Introduc

Chronic Lymphocytic Leukaemia (CLL)

It's bad news if you or a member of your family has CLL. The good news is that there are lots of things we can do to live well, and living well can prolong your life. Generally speaking, CLL is contracted by those of us in our later years but we still want to get the best out of life.

I have CLL. At the time of writing, I have suffered from CLL for 9 years. So this book is written from personal experience. I decided to write this book after years of living with CLL in isolation from other sufferers of the condition. Having to find things out the hard way prompts me to share some of what I have learnt with other CLL sufferers and their families. One's own family and friends can be a great help but in my case, when I got to know another CLL sufferer and her daughter, I immediately felt less alone . . . and talking to fellow patients in the Haematology Clinic has been very reassuring. Medical personnel can deal with the symptoms and prescribe treatment but they are usually short of time, short of resources and staff, and they are not there when we stumble with exhaustion or face our fears in the night.

So this is something of a self-help guide. The book outlines the condition and its treatment in the early years of the illness and how we can live better by adapting our behaviour, our responses and our diet.

This is NOT a medical book. And this is a book to dip into rather than to read from cover to cover. You do not need all the information all at once! The material looks at the issues in a positive way but it is still a lot of information to take in all at once - don't even try. Choose those elements that have relevance for you just now and leave the rest.

If you suffer from other medical conditions as well as CLL, you will need to discuss with your doctor the relevance of the ideas in this book for you as an individual. We all have our own unique responses to ideas, changes and treatment.

One of the worst aspects of any chronic illness is the feeling of fear and helplessness that it generates. This is so counterproductive that just feeling afraid can make us feel worse than we actually are. Whatever our condition, we can do something to feel better by using knowledge well, taking positive actions, and seeking support from others.

Make the most of the best and the least of the worst.
Robert Louis Stevenson, 1850 – 1894, Scottish writer and poet.

The book has its limitations, of course. I am writing largely for the first phase of the illness - often lasting several years - when we are Outpatients with CLL. I have been ill enough myself to have been admitted for a time as an Inpatient, but as this treatment varies so much for each individual, I leave that aspect for the hospital staff and you to manage as well as you can. Always remember though, that you are part of the hospital team in your own treatment and decision-making.

About this book

A word about my background: I have retired after a lifetime teaching primary children, training teachers and writing books and other publications. I specialised in teaching primary science and the way young children learn. Nevertheless, retired or not, I am unable to contain my curiosity, I can't stop asking questions or trying to find some answers. I recommend the process - ask questions of your doctors and nurses. The more informed we are, the better we are at managing our CLL.

NB. I am not a qualified doctor or dietician. Any medical information included has been checked with qualified doctors/haematologists/pharmacists. The recipes are my own adaptations of known recipes which aim for a healthy lifestyle for anyone. I have concentrated on including those foods which research is beginning to identify as possibly anti-carcinogenic, and thus particularly helpful to those of us with CLL. The anecdotes are from my own experience or from others with CLL or their families.

The book includes:

- **Information about some of the symptoms and treatment**
- **Some positive strategies to manage some of these symptoms and treatment**
- **Recipes - a few healthy ideas offered**
- **Personal anecdotes - to remind us we are not alone**
- **Sayings - to say out loud to ourselves when we need to think something positive**

So, reader, if you or a member of your family suffers from CLL, I greet you with the friendship of someone who knows what you are going through. I hope the book will encourage you to live well with hope and good humour. And the knowledge that any profits from the sale of book will be spent on research to find solutions to healing CLL.

CLL: Not the end of the world

What is CLL?

Chronic lymphocytic leukaemia is a condition in which the lymphocyte cells in our blood (one of our white blood cells - see page 31) begin to grow out of control. In that sense it is a kind of slow-growing cancer. CLL is not like an aggressive tumour which attacks quickly; most of us with CLL live for many years with the condition. We don't know yet what causes CLL but there is no evidence that it is inherited, and it is neither contagious nor infectious.

All living things have cells that normally reproduce themselves healthily as required throughout the life of the whole body. Some cells may suddenly mutate or spontaneously change - we don't know why. Most of these cells don't live and we don't even know these changes have happened. Some spontaneous changes in cells can turn out to be beneficial but some are harmful.

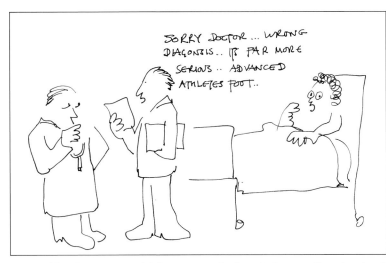

Getting the initial diagnosis

Diagnosis is not always received in a straightforward way. Some patients are diagnosed when they show symptoms of poor immunity to infections, unexplained sensitivity to bruising, excessive exhaustion or anaemia (see page 21). I was diagnosed by accident. My GP gave me a blood test for a skin condition and she picked up a high count of lymphocytes. It took 3 more blood tests, one with her, two at the hospital, to confirm that I suffered from CLL. Whatever the conditions, and whoever confirms the diagnosis, the news can be shocking and upsetting. The word chronic means incurable, and the word leukaemia refers to cancer of the blood.

It can help to have someone with you for the diagnosis and/or subsequent visits to the Haematology Clinic, but many of us have had to do everything alone. My family are very supportive but live all around the world, which has left me to fend for myself. Even with family or friends we can feel helpless - being part of the management of our illness can reduce that feeling of helplessness.

> *Truly, it is in the darkness that one finds the light, so when we are in sorrow, then this light is nearest to us.*
> Johannes Eckhart, c.1260 - 1327, German mystic.

> *When it is dark enough, you can see the stars.*
> Ralph Waldo Emerson, 1803 – 1882, American essayist, poet and philosopher.

What information do you want?

There you are, suddenly informed that you - or a member of your close family - has CLL. This is not necessarily the best time to be given too much information. Furthermore, when we are in that situation, we do not know what is 'too much'. Doctors are busy professionals with other patients waiting, so they may give you a lot of information in a short space of time. They may ask you *'Would you like to know how the disease develops?'* but that still might be too much.

When I was diagnosed, my consultant, with the best of intentions, told me I could hope for another '5-10 years of life'. Coming from a younger man, offering 5-10 years to someone nearly sixty probably seemed like a bonus. After all, it was not as bad as being diagnosed as having an aggressive tumour. Nevertheless, I was shattered. Knowing too much can make us work towards the expectation that doctors have, like a self-fulfilling prophecy. In my case, I felt I was working out a life sentence. It is better to travel forwards hopefully, as a positive approach can actively improve your view of the illness, encourage you to take positive steps for yourself, and prolong your life just that bit more and that bit better.

If you have been given more information than you need right now, store it away in your mind as the 'worst case scenario' and try to forget it for now. You do not have to jump over all the hurdles or deal with all the symptoms today. It might be better if consultants gave only basic information to begin with, preferably reinforced with a written outline for the patient to take away. And the information must be as positive as possible!

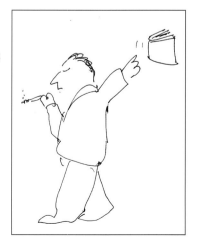

Booklets from the best cancer organisations may also give us too much information too soon. Information obtained on the Internet can be extensive and prove very distressing. You may find out the whole progress of the disease in one fell swoop - very depressing! Even leaflets included with medication, legally required to give as much information as possible, can be daunting. Of course, it is necessary to provide information for people with conditions other than CLL, e.g. pregnancy, diabetes, high cholesterol, etc. We all need to know about possible side effects of treatment, but reading about the more extreme effects can be scary. A little information at a time is easier to absorb. Hospital pharmacists can be very helpful in giving us a positive perspective on side effects of medication.

If you feel overloaded with information, ask for an appointment with your consultant when you and a friend can talk to him/her, with a set of questions that you want answered that deal with your situation at this time. **And only read the chapters of this book that are relevant to your situation right now** - leave the rest for another time. You might not need some of it at all.

Some information can be very basic, such as simple changes to our diet. A medical journalist suggested aiming for a diet that is a *'rainbow of fruit and vegetables'*. Such a rainbow of colours gives a variety of vitamins and minerals: reds (beetroot, raspberries), oranges (oranges, peppers, carrots, etc.), greens, yellows, purples, whites. The information made choices and planning meals so much easier to remember.

Making plans

Don't make drastic changes in your life too soon. You will need time to come to terms with the implications of the CLL but if you have been diagnosed early, your life will probably not change much to begin with. I personally carried on working full-time for nearly two years and part-time for another three years before I really had to cut down on the exacting demands of work. Pace yourself!

It is not only important for the family to be aware of the symptoms of CLL, but at times you will need to enlist their help and understanding. One of the positive aspects of CLL is that we can look healthy a lot of the time. The downside is that friends and family can easily forget that we need more care than pre-CLL. We get exhausted more easily, we may lack energy, particularly during treatment. We need to pace ourselves and find the balance between exertion and taking exercise and giving ourselves time to recover. It is not comfortable to get run down.

> *To keep a lamp burning we have to keep putting oil in it.*
> Mother Theresa of Calcutta, 1910 – 1997, Yugoslav-born missionary.

Then our friends and family need reminders that our immunity is compromised, severely so during treatment. As far as possible we need to avoid being in close contact with people who have colds, flu and other infections. This can be distressing but it is better than catching an infection that takes weeks from which to recover.

> *I once had to avoid my daughter and grandchildren for 4 weeks whilst chicken pox worked its way through. It was difficult at the time, but the subsequent get-together when everyone was free from infection was all the happier.*

There are things we can take to minimise infections - check with your GP, consultant or herbalist (see references). We may look slightly paranoid to some people who are less close to us, but stick to your guns. If you have to visit someone who is sick, keep some distance between you and/or wear a hygienic mask (available from good pharmacies), and always wash your hands thoroughly with a good antiseptic soap afterwards. You will be a

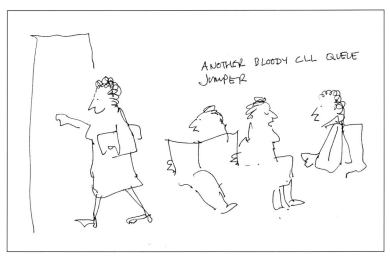

priority for flu vaccinations each autumn - ask your GP about this. You may be entitled to other vaccinations against TB and other illnesses, but always check with your GP and consultant as to what is best for you.

Symptoms and strategies to manage them

What symptoms might you experience?

In the early stages of the illness, you may experience no symptoms or very few. Subsequently, you may experience some of the following in response to the illness and the medication:

- Tiredness and breathlessness
- Low immunity to infections, frequent and/or prolonged infections
- Swollen glands/lymph nodes
- Fluctuating temperatures, fever and sweating
- Bruising and bleeding
- Sleeplessness
- Anaemia
- Weight loss or weight gain
- Diarrhoea
- Hair thinning or hair loss
- Low blood pressure - feeling faint

Feelings

We feel a range of feelings, such as disbelief, fear, distress, a sense of loss, uncertainty, helplessness, anger, unfairness (why me?) and concern for our dependent or extended family. In that dreadful moment, we often stop being a person and become a patient with CLL. This sudden reversal of who we are, our identity, can undermine our strength and ability to ask questions or ask for help.

It may be that close members of your family have their own troubles and you don't wish to upset them. This can be a heavy responsibility on top of the shock of the diagnosis. In my case, I was mostly upset for my daughter - I know that it was enormously difficult for her to come to terms with my illness. We all have feelings throughout the course of the illness as we see-saw through treatment and remission, through symptoms and their effects on us. But we can survive these if we accept them and allow people to help us.

And in the sweetness of friendship, let there be laughter, and sharing of pleasures. For in the dew of little things the heart finds its morning and is refreshed.

Khalil Gibran, 1883 – 1931, Lebanese poet, artist and mystic.

Who can help?

You will know what is best for you but I suggest it is essential that you are able to talk to someone about the CLL, whether with family or professionals. Talking about it can help us regain our status as persons and give us a more positive perspective, as well as strategies to manage our lives better.

> At the start of my illness, I thought I could cope more or less by myself. However, later that year, I travelled to Australia to see two of my brothers. On the way from the airport I began to talk openly and just broke down, distressing for my family but ultimately a great release for my feelings.

Organisations

There are no organisations at this time that are set up exclusively for those of us suffering from CLL and our families. Perhaps they will exist in the future but there may be some resistance. I tried and failed to set up such a group in my own hospital - you might have more luck than I did. There are general bodies that offer support or counselling to sufferers from all types of leukaemia and cancer, such as LEUKAEMIA CARE and CANCERBACUP (see page 65 for details)

Both organisations have offices and/or regional teams around the UK and offer a variety of useful booklets addressing many aspects of cancer and its treatment. Although the booklets are written for all types of leukaemia or cancer, much of what is written in them has direct application for those of us with CLL.

Counsellors

Most GP's surgeries and hospitals have full-time counsellors, but on your first diagnosis they are unlikely to be there, and their services may not even be offered. Even when they are offered, we can be too shocked to see them anyway, so another visit to the hospital is necessary.

Some of us hide our feelings more successfully, and consultants may perceive this as 'a good sign' and deal with us clinically rather than personally, thus emphasising that we are now patients not persons. We have to recover ourselves. We are still persons, albeit persons with an illness, an illness we can manage and maybe live with for many years. Always remember, you are a person, not just Patient No. 12345!

> Live all you can: it's a mistake not to. It doesn't matter what you do in particular, so long as you have had your life. If you haven't had that, what have you had?
> Henry James, 1843 - 1916, American novelist.

Tiredness and breathlessness

If you are in the very early stages of CLL, you may not experience any real difficulties between your levels of energy pre-diagnosis and now. As the disease develops, CLL sufferers tend to experience an increased susceptibility to tiredness. Climbing stairs and other forms of exertion or activity can become more difficult as time goes on.

Changes in energy levels can be difficult to measure, as many of us with CLL are also getting older and might normally experience a loss of energy. Nevertheless, we are likely to become even more fatigued than others without CLL. This may be worse if we become anaemic (see page 21). However, we can do a great deal to manage life well and minimise the effects of fatigue.

NB. If you experience severe breathlessness, do not hesitate in consulting your GP or your Haematologist - it is important to catch infections such as chest or gastric infections early on. Our low immunity and some of the medication we have to take makes us vulnerable, and we do not want infections to develop into something more serious.

What positive strategies can we use?

- Start practising daily deep breathing in a relaxed way. It will calm you and help your intake of oxygen too. Get into a good habit and use your deep breathing whenever you might need extra oxygen - going upstairs, dealing with a problem, waiting to see your consultant, having a blood test. Join a yoga class or Pilates or similar. These teach good relaxation as well as good breathing techniques, and strengthen our hearts, lungs and other muscles.

- Look at your general life schedule to see where changes can be made to reduce any tiredness or fatigue. For example, try to pace your commitments to work, family and friends. You now have an excellent excuse to take things easier. Limit how many things you try to achieve each week or each day. Follow a busy day with a quiet evening at home, follow an energetic day with the family with a quiet day or two, follow a holiday spent travelling with a very relaxing week or two at home. If receiving treatment, plan your day to do little jobs with frequent rests in between.

- Take exercise in ways that you enjoy. Take walks, join yoga or other classes, swim, join a Line Dancing class. Being active helps us to sleep better too. The secret is to enjoy yourself and keep fit whilst not overdoing it. If you feel tired, sit out, sit down, stop and rest. Walking is always good and you can easily limit how much you can manage.

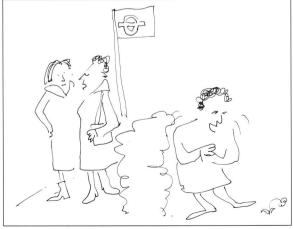

- If you are in a class, make sure the teacher knows about your condition and how you feel on the day.

    My own yoga teacher redesigns aspects of the work for me as an individual (all good teachers will do this), enables me to succeed without overdoing it and encourages me to adopt resting positions during the class. My fellow class-mates are friendly and understanding.

- Watch or listen to funny shows on DVD, radio or TV, read funny books, see theatre comedies. Laughter has always been called 'the best medicine' and research is beginning to show that there are positive medical changes inside us when we laugh on a regular basis. If you are often alone (as I am), try smiling at yourself, smile at the garden or the birds in the air. Make pretend and laugh out loud with a Ha! Ha! Ha! There is even evidence that pretend laughter has a positive effect on our bodies. How about that!

  Don't wait for a light to appear at the end of the tunnel, stride down there . . . and light the bloody thing yourself.
  Sara Henderson, b.1936, Australian Outback Station Manager and writer.

- Make a list of the things you wanted to do but 'never had the time'. This could be reading more books, joining an evening class or a local U3A daytime group (University of the Third Age, see page 67), take up photography or singing, bowling or join a Book Club. Since the start of my CLL I have done folk-dancing, met great people in U3A on some fascinating museum projects, started drawing and gone back to singing after 20 years!

- Indulge yourself if and whenever you can. Feeling good about yourself helps you to manage the illness and live more positively. Buy that extra-warm coat for the winter months or that special garden feature. Have a nice hairdo or massage. Have occasional or regular treatments or therapies that make you feel good, such as reflexology, aromatherapy, swimming. Always make sure that professionals are aware of your condition and the implications.

  Since my diagnosis, I have gone up in a hot-air balloon (something I always wanted to do), had aromatherapy and reflexology.

- Obtain additional advice or help from alternative therapists or healers, such as herbalists or people in your church, temple or mosque.

  I have gone to healing centres and although no miracles occurred, these have been positive encounters that helped me keep a positive perspective on things.

- Schedule time for interesting activities but put limitations on the demands of these, such as playing with grandchildren or travelling abroad. You can accomplish a great deal with good planning and care. For example, visit the family or have them visit you when they are free from infection and put reasonable limits on how long you spend together. Regular, short visits will tire you less than more prolonged visits. I cannot say I always get this right myself. I am impatient and independent and have often overdone things and been exhausted the following day. With practice, you will find out how much you can do in a day, and either stop at the right time, or decide to carry on but allow for an extended rest period the following day or two. Find your own balance.

- Consider your resting environment. Look around your living room or bedroom, and think what changes you might make to have a positive environment in which to spend and enjoy your time. Add something colourful, since warm colours can make us feel more cheerful; pictures or photographs which will remind you of loving family and make you smile; a comfortable chair positioned so you can look out over the garden, perhaps with a pair of binoculars so you can watch the wildlife there.

- Make sure you have all necessary vaccinations well before travelling and obtain appropriate travel insurance (See Finance section). Always check in advance with your GP and consultant before booking visits abroad.

- Take a folding, portable seat with you (e.g. The National Trust sell two or three types) and carry it with you everywhere (or persuade a friend to carry it). Use for a quick rest in the street, the station concourse, in museums and stately homes. Airlines will let you take the folding seat with you, either as cabin luggage, stored in a steward's locker, or sent in the luggage hold.

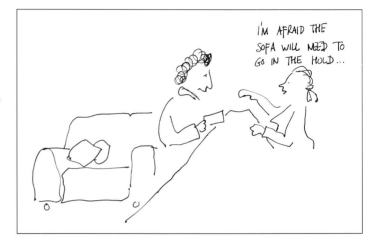

Since the onset of my CLL, I have finally visited Macchu Picchu in Peru and the pyramids of Egypt, all with the magic aid of my folding chair. Even the most able-bodied on those trips envied me my ever-ready rest-chair!

- Eat for health! You need a good regular diet with energy foods, with vitamins and minerals and possibly extra iron. Check with your GP and haematologist before embarking on the latter. Try out some of the recipes at the end of the book.

Low immunity to infections, frequent and/or prolonged infections

We want to keep as well as we can, whether during treatment or remission periods. There is truth in the adage that *Prevention is better than cure*. Avoiding infections is one area you will have to begin disciplining yourself quite carefully. CLL reduces our immunity to infections. We are vulnerable. Our low level of immunity means that we cannot fight infections effectively, we do not have the same resistance and some of the medication can reduce our immunity even further. For example, a bad cold that lasts 4-5 days with your friends may last 2-3 weeks for you and me and feel much more severe. You may have a persistent cough that lasts for a few weeks after that.

What positive strategies can we use?

- Much as you love your friends and family, you and they will have to stay out of reach if they have an infection. This can be very difficult and sometimes distressing to stick to, but your health is vitally important. After a while your family and friends not only become very understanding, but will be the first to postpone meetings when they might expose you to infection by close contact. This is their way of showing consideration and affection. Cuddling shows affection, but you are vulnerable and have low immunity.

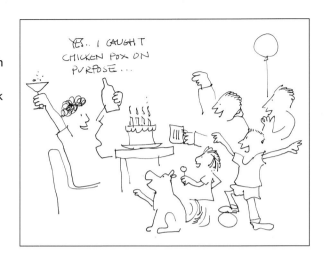

- Get into a habit of washing your hands more frequently and more thoroughly with a good antiseptic soap, when preparing meals, after gardening (even if you wear gardening gloves), after contact with children who may have mild infections.

- Keep a supply of hygienic masks, available from any good pharmacist, so that if close family and friends suffering from infections really want or need to see you, they can slip one of these on and visit you whilst reducing the risk of infecting you too.

- Consult your GP immediately for help in reducing infections when you notice symptoms such as a high temperature, a sore throat, diarrhoea, etc. An immediate response to an infection is better than waiting for it to develop into something harder to shift. If your doctor (or herbalist) recommends medication, try to store some at home so that you can begin the fight against an infection as soon as you recognise it, even on a Sunday or Bank Holiday when pharmacies may be closed.

- If you need to travel, consult your GP and consultant about which vaccines you should and should not have. For example, if you are receiving chemotherapy, you should not be given 'live virus' vaccines such as those for polio or measles. Other vaccines may be appropriate, such as those for tetanus, hepatitis A, hepatitis B, cholera, etc. It is important to check well in advance. There is a vaccination against pneumonia you could qualify for, and you will also be a priority for flu vaccinations each autumn. Ask your GP about this.

- Herbalists and homeopaths can be very helpful in advising you of alternative remedies. There is some scepticism amongst traditional medical personnel about these therapies, but it is always worth trying alternative therapies - you might be one of the people for whom these therapies work. My own herbalist has been invaluable in helping me cope with infections when they have arisen, as well as giving me lots of positive time to talk!

- To a certain extent, going out on public transport and attending public events can also be a risk, but with care and good luck, we don't usually catch too many infections that way. Watch out for the insensitive people in the cinema or theatre who are obviously infectious and/or coughing openly too near you, and keep out of their way.

- Make positive changes to your diet. Examples are included later in the book. Additionally, when you are feeling energetic, make double quantities of a meal and freeze half for another day. Allow friends and family to prepare some meals for you - tell them what you can easily prepare and enjoy eating, and give them the recipes at the end of this book too.

- You may want to seek out a registered healer, whether you have a religious faith or not. Some people gain considerable comfort from such visits, whether or not the symptoms are reduced.

  We are all travellers in the wilderness of this world, and the best we can find in our travels is an honest friend.
  Robert Louis Stevenson, 1850 – 1894, Scottish writer and poet.

- Take a fresh look at your bedlinen and pillows. We all have bed mites which can contribute to stuffy breathing. Frequent washing (at 50°C) kills some of these off but it is worth considering more frequent replacing of your pillows and drycleaning of duvets. Apart from refreshing the linen, this can cheer us up too!

Swollen glands/swollen lymph nodes

Swollen glands occur when the excess lymphocyte cells collect together, generally in the lymph nodes (the junctions of the lymphatic system) located in the neck, in the armpits, in the groin and the spleen. Their function is to drain excess tissue fluid into the veins. Quite often, the glands may swell up but go down again after an infection. These swollen glands are often painless but can sometimes cause pain and discomfort. Over time, some of the glands will remain swollen permanently. On the whole we must rely on our doctors to monitor the increase of lymphocytes and take action to reduce these whenever it becomes necessary. We cannot halt the overall progress of swollen glands or the spleen, but we can have a positive effect on slowing their growth.

What positive strategies can we use?

- We can reduce the frequency of swollen glands by avoiding as many infections as we can. CLL sufferers are more prone to catch infections such as colds and flu and other diseases. We are what is known as immuno-compromised. Reducing the incidence of infections throughout the year can slow the development of swelling lymph nodes. (See Infections: Positive strategies above.)

- Ask your GP or hospital dietician to suggest appropriate prescriptions or medications you can buy over the counter in the pharmacy that you can take immediately when you catch an infection. Shortening an infection period will positively influence your glands. An immediate response to an infection is better than waiting for it to develop.

- Herbalists and other alternative therapists can often supply you with ideas to respond promptly to the onset of an infection. Consult registered, qualified therapists who will have experience in advising you of remedies.

- Increase the range and number of fruit and vegetables in your diet. These should be a constant in your daily diet. Fruit and vegetables are known to give us some defence against infections, so we might escape becoming infected or reduce its impact.

  If you include a lot of dairy produce in your diet, consider replacing dairy products with soya products. Current research suggests that soya products may have a positive, possibly anti-carcinogenic, effect on our bodies. Try replacing some dairy milk with soya milk or rice milk, try soya yogurts and tofu dishes, non-dairy ice-cream, lower-fat cheeses. If you change to soya products, remember to increase your calcium intake, e.g. by including more meat and green vegetables in your diet. As with everything, do not overdo calcium supplements - too much calcium is not desirable.

  It is only anecdotal evidence, but in my own case the incidence of swollen neck glands has gone down considerably since reducing dairy milk and cheese and adding soya products, such as tofu and soya milk.

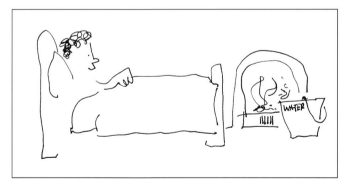

Fluctuating temperatures, fever and sweating

We are often subject to sudden, unexpected changes in temperature, whether during treatment or remission. These typically occur at night but quite often occur during the day as well. The changes in temperature do not usually last long but can be accompanied by massive sweating, followed by rapid cooling when skin and clothes become wet with perspiration. When they occur at night they can cause sleeplessness and distress (see page 19). Whenever they occur, these sudden fevers can be uncomfortable, disconcerting and embarrassing.

What positive strategies can we use?

- Accept that your temperature will fluctuate. Acceptance makes us more positive psychologically and may even reduce the frequency or period of time the fevers last.

- Make sure your friends and family know about this symptom. They will become used to the suddenness of the changes and a) will not draw undue attention to your sudden disrobing and b) offer support by maintaining a suitable household temperature for your benefit. It can even become something to smile about ... "Here we go again!"

The best way to cheer yourself up is to cheer someone else up.
Mark Twain, 1835 – 1910, American writer and humourist.

- Try adapting your clothing so you have layers that can be removed or replaced easily. A soft waistcoat is easier to remove in public than a vest! A loose fleecy jacket can come off quickly to cool down, and go on again quickly enough to stop any uncomfortably rapid cooling.

- Try using 'High-Wick' underwear which allows sweat to pass through, leaving the skin fairly dry. Buy these from sports shops or from on-line skiwear suppliers. Other than that, cotton clothing absorbs the sweat quickly and also dries out quickly.

- With practice, you will begin to recognise the onset of such sudden fevers. When one is starting, quickly undo the top buttons of your blouse or shirt and ease your collar. This will give your body a bit of air. You may not stop the high temperature or sweating from developing but it may peak at a lower level.

- Keep a couple of damp flannels with you in a small plastic bag, whether going out or at night. When you feel a hot temperature or sweat starting up, wrap one of the damp flannels around the back of your neck and use the other to damp your hands and forehead. This can stop the worst of the sweat developing. The cold flannels can be a bit of a shock, but better than being wet with sweat, then cold as the sweat evaporates from your skin and body. If you use flannels regularly, wash them each night in a dilute solution of antiseptic liquid to keep them hygienic.

- **Always carry a bottle of water with you.** You will need to drink more anyway. Additionally, if you recognise the onset of a sudden sweat, take a few sips of water immediately. This may not stop the fever developing, but may limit the period it lasts and lower the peak level. I have learned to do this everywhere, even surreptitiously and unnoticed during dramatic moments in the theatre!

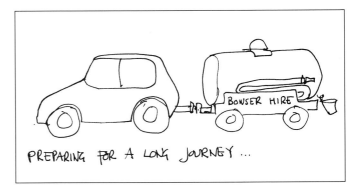

PREPARING FOR A LONG JOURNEY ...

- Even without the sweats, try to drink about 2 litres per day - equivalent to about 8 cups of water, tea, orange juice, etc. Don't get dehydrated!

- Try to maintain a balanced temperature in your bedroom. It is more difficult to cool down following a night fever if the room is too warm. Higher summer temperatures in the UK nowadays make some nights more uncomfortable for all of us, and it is less easy to control this. When too hot, turn down your duvet or blanket quickly until the high peak subsides. Some people find it effective to use a cooling fan on a timer to bring the room temperature down during the middle hours of the night. When the nights are too cold, rapid cooling can take us to the other extreme. I recommend using an oil-filled heater on a timer in your bedroom, timed to come on for a short period during the coldest hours. These heaters are almost silent and can be adjusted to maintain a comfortable room temperature, without making it too warm when you experience a fever. (See Sleeplessness below)

- For some women who are experiencing the menopause or are post-menopausal, the CLL fevers and sweats can exaggerate an existing condition. Try using (with the advice of your doctor and herbalist) soya-isoflavone regularly. You can buy these under that name or as 'Red Clover' tablets. Taking these regularly can help reduce the frequency and scale of the fevers and sweats. Even long after the menopause, soya-isoflavone tablets can help reduce the frequency of the hot sweating.

Bruising and bleeding

When we bump into something, the blood vessels in that part of the body are temporarily damaged. Injured or dead cells have to be removed and new tissue has to be rebuilt. For those of us with CLL, it just takes rather longer for this removal and rebuilding, as there is often a reduction in the healing blood cells (platelets) that respond to bruises and cuts. During the time of recovery from the bruises, we may experience swelling, tenderness and the characteristic colours of bruising.

You may be surprised by the number of small or medium sized bruises you find. We can get bruises from bumps and scrapes against objects that we scarcely noticed happening. Someone may grab our arm enthusiastically or give us a big hug, a beloved grandchild may give us an accidental hit - all pleasurable events, but they can leave us bruised. Similarly, cuts and scrapes may take longer to heal. It is virtually impossible to avoid bruising and minor cuts but there are some measures you can take to manage these better.

What positive strategies can we use?

- First, try to accept that this will happen regularly and try not to worry about it.

- Tell people that you bruise easily. Family, friends, professionals providing treatment, yoga teachers, etc. should know. No-one can prevent bruises and injuries completely, but, on the whole, everyone will take more care of you.

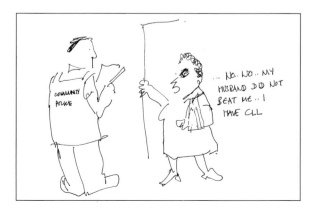

- Go round your house or flat and look for potential hazards that you might bump into or things with sharp edges. Get into a habit of tucking away things that jut out or are left lying around. Persuade your family to join you in this. If you have furniture with particularly sharp edges, consider buying clip-on corner mounts used by families with young toddlers and try these.

- Make some changes in your diet (see page 49). And eat more rutin. It seems to have some effect in reducing the worst of the bruising (see page 51).

- If you receive too much pressure or get a bump that will result in a bruise, massage the area gently straightaway. Arnica has a reputation for reducing bruises. As soon as you have the opportunity, apply a dilute solution of arnica or arnica cream to the area (available from pharmacies) and repeat the applications until the bruise goes down. There is no real way to reduce the bruise substantially but the arnica may reduce the swelling a bit.

- If you have a minor cut or injury, deal with it straightaway. Cuts that are clean and covered give the clotting cells the best environment to begin the healing process quickly. Clean the area and if necessary apply a plaster or other dressing. Use an antiseptic cream where necessary. Major injuries should be dealt with by medical personnel in the usual way.

- Experiment with different plasters. The best plasters for those of us with CLL are not only sterile, they stick without subsequent discomfort and even more bruising when we remove them. Look for children's or allergenic plasters which cover cuts but do not pull on the skin on removal.

- If your platelet level goes very low, your consultant may advise you to have a platelet transfusion (see page 32).

Sleeplessness

You may experience periods of sleeplessness during the night, from changing temperatures and sweating, or anxieties and concerns, or some other discomfort and symptoms. Then the sleeplessness itself becomes the problem. We all begin to worry that we will be too tired to manage the following day's activities, etc. The whole thing can become a vicious circle.

What positive strategies can we use?

- First and foremost, it is best to accept that it will happen. Psychologically, that makes us relax more when it does happen and helps us to go back to sleep more quickly.

- Deal with symptoms such as sudden fever or sweating (see page 16). Wear loose, comfortable clothing and use easy to remove bedlinen so you can cool down and warm up again quickly.

- Being reasonably active during the day can help to give you some extended periods of sleep in between periods of sleeplessness.

- Develop a night-time ritual so that winding down to sleep becomes part of the programme - e.g. a bath, a warm drink, reading a few pages of a book.

- Position a radio, tape recorder or CD player beside your bed. Use tapes or CDs of quiet, enjoyable music and audio stories during the night to distract you from becoming anxious, from being overly conscious of your heart rate or fast pulse, from your fears and anxieties. It is possible that you will fall asleep during the story, but the great thing about using a CD or audio-tape is that you simply rewind or reload and listen to it properly another time.

  This has become such a part of my programming that sometimes I have barely begun to listen to the tape before I fall asleep, and I don't even hear the tape switch off.

- The World Service on the BBC is on throughout the night but is not necessarily always a positive thing to listen to. World news can bring all the unhappiness of the world right into your bedroom. However, the World Service also includes many interesting programmes too, so it is always worth giving that station a try, along with other stations.

- Try using a self-hypnosis CD or audio tape. Buy from a good health food store or buy online from a reputable website. These are not intended to put you into a deep hypnotic state, but calm you down so that you drift off to sleep. They may not work too well if you are in pain, but is very relaxing when anxieties are troubling you and preventing you from sleeping. If you feel that you need greater support than self-hynosis, ask whether your hospital has a hypnotherapist who can give you this help, or look for reputable established hypnotherapists who have independent practices. They may be expensive, but can be worth their fees. If you are in pain for some reason, ask your consultant to refer you to the Pain Management Surgeon in your hospital. It is remarkable how much relief and comfort can be prescribed to help reduce any particular pain you may have.

- After a poor night's sleep, try to plan an afternoon nap or even a quiet sit-down with your eyes closed after lunch. A short break then can give you another burst of energy to manage the rest of the day and evening.

- Make your last meal early enough so that your digestive system is not working full-time late at night. Keep the meal light if possible, with only moderate drinking of alcohol. This is not an absolute rule. When we are eating with friends and family, it is not appropriate to impose our rules on them, although they may already be adjusting to your schedule.

Anaemia

Red blood cells are the cells that collect oxygen from the blood vessels in the lungs and carry it around the body. This oxygen reacts with sugars and starches stored in muscles to release energy and carbon dioxide. The oxygen-depleted blood carries the carbon dioxide back to the blood vessels in the lungs, to be discharged there when we breathe out. The red blood cells then collect more oxygen to transport around the body. This constant release of energy is necessary to maintain our body temperature, to keep our organs operating properly, keep our hearts pumping, our lungs breathing, our brains thinking and our muscles moving.

When we are anaemic, we might be short of red blood cells because they are not being produced in sufficient quantity by the bone marrow. We might have an iron deficiency, or the red blood cells might not be functioning effectively due to treatment. The effects that are most noticeable to us are likely to be lack of energy and tiredness, or getting cramps frequently. This can be very distressing. We may also lack concentration, we feel reluctant to make the effort to socialise, and even the most basic chores feel like mountain-climbing.

What positive strategies can we use?

- Diet is important. You need a balanced diet with a satisfactory intake of foods containing iron. Eat with moderation. For example, eggs contain iron but can also raise cholesterol levels and cause constipation; spinach contains iron but also a lot of oxalic acid; rocket and watercress are good but too much can cause diarrhoea, etc. As usual, consult your doctor or consultant or herbalist for advice.

- You may be advised by your doctor or dietician or herbalist to take supplementary iron as well. Health food shops and pharmacies can supply you with liquid iron formulas (e.g. Fluorodix) or tablets. Digesting is probably easier with the liquid formula but as this has to be kept refrigerated, having tablets is a convenient form of supply too. Do follow the instructions given by your GP, therapist and on the packet.

- Try to give some responsibility for making decisions to partners or family. Removing some of the stress of decision-making reduces demands on your energy and allows you to concentrate your energies on what is important.

- Stay as positive as you can whenever you can!

  With our thoughts we make the world.
  Buddha, c.563 - 483 BC, Indian religious teacher and founder of Buddhism.

- For other strategies, follow the ideas listed under Tiredness above to pace yourself and get help.

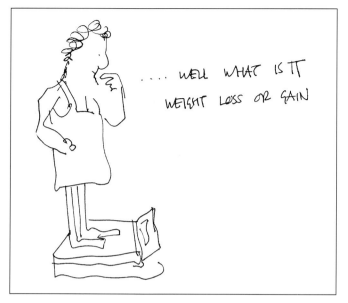

Weight loss or weight gain

During the early stages of CLL, if you are on medication such as chemotherapy and have no other health conditions, your weight is likely to remain stable. Changes can occur when we become ill or we are prescribed treatment. Steroids, for example, can make us feel hungry even when we do not really need to eat, so we put on weight. Some treatments make us lose our appetite, cause sickness or diarrhoea, and so we lose weight.

All this can have an effect on how we feel. We spend many years building identity, not least in how we appear to ourselves in the mirror. Whilst we are not always satisfied with our appearance, any changes, particularly changes over which we have limited control, can be distressing. We may feel less recognisable as ourselves, embarrassed, less attractive, uncomfortable with family and friends or strangers and even want to avoid seeing people or have them see us.

I experienced all these feelings when put on a high steroid treatment. The condition is known colloquially by medical staff as 'Moonface'. My swollen cheeks distorted my face, my mouth and eyes. I looked like a fat hamster - even my dimples disappeared! I felt distressed and not like myself at all. Fortunately, people around me were positive (especially the grandchildren, who didn't even notice!) and the condition went down as the dosage was eventually reduced.

What positive strategies can we use?

- Talk about your feelings with friends, family, your doctor, a dietician, a counsellor.

- Trust that the people who care about you will support you. You are still the person they know and love.

  One word frees us of all the weight and pain of life: that word is love.
  Sophocles, 496 - 406 BC, Greek tragedian.

- Talk to a dietician at the hospital or your GP's surgery.

- Plan your diet carefully. Try eating smaller portions more frequently and regularly.

- If you feel hungry for sweet things, eat fruit instead of biscuits or cake. It won't always work but when it does, we gain in confidence instead of gaining weight!

- Some treatments can cause constipation and you may be prescribed laxatives as well as other medication. You might be able to cut down on the laxatives if you add foods such as sunflower seeds and dried fruit, particularly apricots, prunes, dried apples and peaches. These stimulate the gut to work harder and reduce the need for medication.

- Always maintain a high fluid intake. You can vary the fluids for interest: filtered water, sparkling mineral water, apple or orange juice, herbal teas, especially those which may have a positive effect on your digestion, such as root ginger, ginger and lemon, peppermint, camomile, and so on (see page 59 for Smoothies). Never forget - don't leave home without your bottle of water!

- When you have the energy, make double quantities of a meal and freeze half so you have something available for those days when you can't face cooking a meal.

- Allow friends and family to prepare some meals for you. Sometimes family need to have something tangible to do to feel supportive, and this will make them feel valued and purposeful.

Diarrhoea

We are more likely to be subject to diarrhoea due to both the CLL and treatment. Diarrhoea can be uncomfortable, painful, distressing and embarrassing. It can affect many aspects of our lives, not least when we want to socialise with family and friends or live an active life. Diarrhoea can reduce our energy levels still further, and deprive us of the nutrition we need to live well.

Diarrhoea needs treating quickly. We may also have been prescribed antibiotics as part of our more general medication which trigger diarrhoea by killing off friendly, beneficial bacteria in the intestines or colon, one of the side effects that we have to cope with and overcome.

What positive strategies can we use?

- Let your GP and consultant know. They may wish to test for gastric infections and prescribe appropriate medication. They will recommend something (e.g. Loperamide) which will give temporary relief whilst they diagnose the problem.

- Never underestimate how much you need to drink. You need lots of fluids - 2 litres per day! Carry a bottle of water around with you and keep sipping in between meals.

- You may need to change your diet temporarily. Avoid or reduce some of the more fibrous foods, such as grains, fresh fruit. Substitute with a diet of smaller but more frequent meals. Include more easily digestible foods, such as chicken, white fish, plain breads and cereals rather than granary bread or wholewheat pasta or rice. Stewed or tinned fruit is easier on the digestion than fresh fruit, although bananas are said to be 'binding'. Avoid spicy or fatty foods. Find foods that work for you as an individual, as that will mean you will enjoy eating.

- Root ginger can have a preventative effect on reducing the symptoms of diarrhoea, such as discomfort or pain. Ginger can be ingested in many pleasant ways. Include it in soup, stir-fries, herbal teas, or buy it as crystallised ginger.

- Some medication may cause constipation. Usually your doctor or consultant will prescribe additional medication to counteract the constipation effects. However, one way of reducing the reliance on laxatives is to increase your intake of nuts (unless allergic), seeds and dried fruits. Stores and supermarkets sell packets of nuts and raisins and dried fruit mixes which are really tasty and effective. Take a few of these twice a day.

Hair thinning or hair loss

Although we may be in the early stages of CLL, and even with initial treatment by the first type of chemotherapy (e.g. Chlorambucil), most of us do not suffer hair loss. As chemotherapy treatment becomes more aggressive, some of us do suffer hair loss or our hair stops growing. This is distressing. Hair is such a big part of our identity, and thinning or hair loss can make us feel older, frail and embarrassed. This might feel worse if you have not been warned in advance. You may not be told that treatment with more toxic chemotherapy such as fludarabine or cyclophosphomide, is likely to produce hair loss or thinning. This may not be as severe as patients who are treated with radiotherapy, but it is still distressing when it happens. Our hair will grow again, but not necessarily in such abundance as it did before treatment.

What positive strategies can we use?

- Initially, you may not wish to act. Just wait and see where and how your hair grows.

- Extend the periods between haircuts or postpone haircuts temporarily.

- Use gentle shampoo less frequently, and try shampoos + conditioners. Dry your hair using low-level heat from your hairdryer.

- Avoid strong hair treatments like dyes, perms, bleaches, etc.

- Consider changing your hairstyle to accommodate your new appearance.

- Men might wish to avoid wet shaving and use an electric shaver. This might also help to avoid cuts or bruising.

- Wear a high-block sun factor and hat if you go out in the sun, to prevent your skin burning and more damage to the hair follicles.

- Don't dismiss the importance of wigs. Nowadays specialist hairdressers supply and trim wigs for cancer and radiotherapy patients, which can enhance our appearance and look real. Ask at your hospital for local suppliers.

Low blood pressure - feeling faint

Our blood pressure fluctuates during the day and varies according to how active we are. Treatment can trigger changes in our normal pattern and greater fluctuations in blood pressure. One effect of low blood pressure is that we feel faint or dizzy when we sit up or stand up suddenly.

What positive strategies can we use?

- Practise deep slow breathing on a regular basis. Breathe in slowly through your nose and breathe out gently through your mouth. Do this regularly.

- Learn to move more slowly. Don't move too fast when you get up from sitting or lying down. Go upstairs slowly, breathing slowly and deeply. Don't hurry for anything if you can manage it.

- Try to keep your anxiety levels low. Planning in advance for periods when you will have to exert yourself (e.g. visiting the hospital for blood tests) can help to reduce stress. Have things ready in advance, and in the Haematology Clinic ask for a choice of consultation times - not always possible but you might find a degree of flexibility allows you to choose a time more convenient to your schedule.

- Practise laughing out loud, even if it is pretend laughter. There is some evidence to suggest that even pretend laughter increases the antitoxins in our blood, and laughter makes us breathe more deeply too.

- Talk to friends and family, person to person or on the telephone. Apart from making us feel better, talking makes us breathe more deeply and can restore our blood pressure to a more normal level.

Blood Tests

What is a blood test?

Before each meeting with your haematologist you will have a blood test to provide information on your current condition. This is a small sample of blood usually taken from the vein in one of your elbows or somewhere else on one of your arms. You will need to have blood tests from now on for the rest of your life. For some people, this will be relatively easy. A tourniquet is applied which raises a chosen vein, a needle is inserted and a small amount of blood is withdrawn. Many people will feel virtually no pain. Sometimes, and depending on the expertise of the blood technicians, there will be some scarring on the veins from the frequency of the blood tests.

For those of us who are afraid of needles or seeing blood or have a low pain threshold, the blood tests can be one of the worst aspects of CLL. In my own case, for 4 years I was more afraid of the Blood Room than I was of each new diagnosis. Four years of distress before I discovered methods of positive action to allay my fears and reduce the discomfort.

Sometimes your consultant will ask for additional small samples of blood for other tests and for research purposes. This is all done very simply from the same blood test. If you are asked to give an additional sample for research purposes, do sign this as the research will eventually help to find a solution to the illness.

What happens in a blood test?

During each consultation, you will usually be given a form which allows you to go directly into the Blood Test Room on your next visit. (On other occasions you may be asked to give a blood sample in the Ward dedicated to Haematology Outpatients, where an experienced nurse will take the blood sample). In most hospitals there will be several blood technicians working in the Blood Room. The frequency of your visits and the mobility of hospital staff means that it is unlikely that you will see the same blood technician twice. Although all of the staff are professional, some are more experienced than others.

You will usually take the blood sample directly to the Blood Analysis Lab. You may wait for the analysis print-out, or it may be sent by computer to your consultant. This analysis has to be done in time for your consultant to have it when you see him/her. Other blood samples are dealt with separately. The print-out is then given to you to take to the Haematology Clinic or Ward, to add to your notes prior to your appointment with your consultant.

What positive strategies can we use to manage the pain and discomfort?

● **Local anaesthetic**

Your GP can prescribe a cream, which acts as a local anaesthetic. This is applied to the veins at the elbow, or on the chosen vein in your arm or hand, some time prior to the blood test (read the instructions given by the GP and on the packet). This anaesthetises the localised area over the vein and reduces the pain. The blood technician can remove the plaster for you. If you find that there is discomfort when plasters are ripped off too painfully, you can remove the plaster yourself and wash your elbow just prior to the blood test (stop off in the visitor's toilet before going to the Blood Test Room). The blood technicians will always thoroughly clean the vein area as well.

● **Choice of needle**

You can ask the blood technician to use a *butterfly needle*. This needle has a smaller piercing point and is less painful. It only takes a few seconds longer than the regular needle but it is worth it. The blood technicians are usually happy to co-operate with you in this choice. If you have difficulty, **ask your consultant to specify a butterfly on the request form.** Frequent blood tests in the same place cause scarring and this can make the needle slip. Those of us with CLL are entitled to use strategies that reduce blood loss in the elbow and limit distress or discomfort.

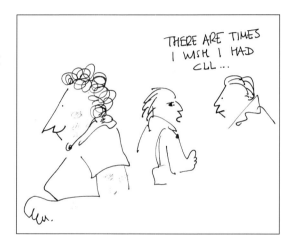

● **Breathing**

When your arm is prepared for the blood test, take a deep breath in and release the breath slowly. This relaxes you and your arm and makes the process much easier.

● **Alternate the arms**

Make a note of which arm is used for each blood test and alternate them for each visit. Blood technicians are happy to oblige with your request to use a chosen arm.

● **Rutin**

Start taking Rutin on a regular basis. Rutin helps to make up the cell tissue of the veins, making the veins stronger and better able to withstand frequent blood tests. There may also be a reduction of bleeding under the skin. Rutin may also reduce the bruising, to which those of us who suffer from CLL are very prone. Rutin is found in the pith of citrus fruits (more tasty than you think!) and can also be bought in tablet form in health food shops and pharmacies. If you regularly include oranges with pith (see recipes below) in your daily diet, you shouldn't need supplementary rutin.

- Make sure that the pressure pad is applied properly. If it is too loose, you could have blood leaking into the surrounding tissue under the skin and end up with a bruise lasting a week or two. A good blood test leaves little other than a small puncture in the skin.

- After the blood test, keep the tested arm straight and comfortable. Avoid bending that arm or carrying something on that arm - either of which is likely to extend the bleeding under the skin and/or cause bruising.

An effective blood test should leave very little or no bleeding under the skin. You won't always know whether this has occurred until an hour or two after the test when you remove the cotton wool and sticky tape. Get into the habit of noting down the name of your blood technician and go and show the result of a poor test to the Blood Room Supervisor or Patients' Help Officer or Hospital Service Manager before you leave the hospital. There is no excuse for ineptitude in blood tests.

You are entitled to expect a high standard of professional behaviour from the blood technicians. A few blood technicians can become blasé about treating us as persons, such as talking and joking over our heads instead of giving us the concentrated care we need. Ask your blood technician politely to continue his or her conversation with others after they have completed your blood test.

Facing it, always facing it. That's the way to get through. Face it.
Joseph Conrad, 1856 - 1924, Polish-born writer.

PS: A note for any blood technicians who may read this

We rely on your help and are grateful for your co-operation in treating us. I am sure that you will enjoy your job even more, and we patients would find the experience more pleasant, if you talk to us as people while you are administering the blood test. Why not say things such as, *'Are you comfortable?'*, *'I will try and make this as painless as I can.'*, *'I think you may have been here before?'*, etc. Ask your managers to give you training in Human Relations as well as Technical Skills if necessary - a positive atmosphere is better for everyone.

Learning to understand the results of your blood test

I think it was Winston Churchill who said 'There are lies, damned lies and statistics'. In a similar way there is data . . . and there is data. Although the results of our blood tests can be compared with medical norms, we all have individual characteristics and we and our consultants will take this into account. Similarly, our current condition will affect the results, for example if we are receiving treatment or are in remission from the illness. Nevertheless, those of us with CLL can interpret some of the information and use it to understand and manage our health more positively.

I am not suggesting that we have the medical expertise to interpret the blood data fully - it requires an experienced haematologist to do that. Our consultants take a host of other information into consideration for their diagnosis and recommendations for treatment, such as the condition of the glands, the spleen, bruising and fevers, etc. However, never forget that you are an important person in the diagnosis and management of your illness. The better you learn how your body reacts to illness and medication, the better informed you are to help in planning the right treatment. We need to look at the norms relative to us as individuals.

For example, in a year of remission, our lymphocyte count may climb higher than any norm until it reaches a level where treatment becomes necessary. During this period, you may generally feel quite well, and manage the fatigue or other symptoms satisfactorily. Then, like me, you may spend several weeks with a haemoglobin level well below the norm but not low enough to require treatment. So you may find it useful to be aware of your own levels and how these are viewed by your own consultant.

> *I was once forced to seek treatment for an infection (low level emergency) in a hospital in another European country. The doctors freaked out at my high level of white blood cells and lymphocytes even though I knew I was in a period of remission. It took me 5 days before they would let me discharge myself!*

What information comes from the blood test
(Remember: Always check the results with your consultant)

The tests carried out by the technicians in the blood testing laboratory are fast and accurate. When collecting the blood test results, you are unlikely to wait more than 10-15 minutes for your blood data. The data is printed out but also stored on the hospital computer for your consultant to access your notes directly. (The computer notes include more details than the print-out we receive.)

Do not try to read the worst case scenario into our results. We need to look at the positive results as well as be realistic. There are normal parameters of good health in our cell counts as follows.

$(10^3$cells / μL = number of cells per volume; g/dL = mass per volume)

Red blood cells (which carry oxygen around the body):
3.5 - 5 ($\times 10^6$ cells / μL)

Haemoglobin (the oxygen-carrying agent in the red blood cells):
12.5 - 17 g/dL (men)
11.5 - 15 g/dL (women)

White blood cells (which fight infection, provide immunity):
Norm = 4 - 11 ($\times 10^3$ cells / μL)

Platelets (in blood plasma, blood clotting agents):
Norm = 140 - 400 ($\times 10^3$ cells / μL)

Neutrophyls: (cells which increase to fight infections):
Norm = 2 - 7 ($\times 10^3$ cells / μL)

Lymphocytes: (cells which normally fight infections):
Norm = 1.5 - 4 ($\times 10^3$ cells / μL)

Some of us find it helpful to keep a record of our results and how we react to treatment. This can help us to see how our body is responding to the treatment or behaving during periods of remission or infection. It gives us a sense of our individuality and provides data and questions to use in discussion with the Haematology Consultant and GP. The record or diary can give us positive feedback and a sense of managing our own illness.

Looking back through my own diary record of the last 8 years, I can compare results year on year. The knowledge that I have survived episodes of high lymphocyte counts and chemotherapy treatment helps me maintain a positive perspective… 'I've done it before, I can do it again!'

In the midst of winter, I finally learned there was in me an invincible summer.
Albert Camus, 1913 - 1960, French writer.

Lymphocyte cells and white blood cells

There are many kinds of lymphocyte cells. They occur in regular blood as one type of our white blood cells and have a life span of 100 - 300 days. Lymphocyte cells normally help to provide specific immune responses, including producing antibodies to combat disease. Individual lymphocytes produce just one kind of antibody so, to protect the body against all types of diseases, we need thousands of different lymphocytes, each capable of recognising and responding to a particular disease. Lymphoid tissue has memory cells so that the reaction to a second exposure to a particular disease can be very rapid, which gives us immunity. This is the basis of vaccinations in children.

Lymphocytes collect in the lymph nodes. Lymph nodes occur at the junctions of the lymphatic system, for example, in the neck, under the armpits and in the groin. Their function is to drain excess tissue fluid into the veins.

It seems a travesty that some of our very own immune cells become rogue cells that multiply out of proportion, such that our immunity is actually compromised! Because they are our own cells, they are not recognised by our bodies as invaders and are therefore not destroyed in the usual way.

The increase in lymphocyte cells means we have relatively lower levels of other vital cells in the blood. For those of us with CLL, the lymphocyte count increases all the time. Eventually, the count approaches a hundred. For example, the data may read: Lymph: 97.64 ($\times 10^3$ cells / μL). At that time, if we haven't already been referred for treatment for some other condition, we will probably be referred for treatment such as chemotherapy. Treatment such as chemotherapy reduces the lymphocytes (and other cells in the blood). Unfortunately, chemotherapy cannot stop the leukaemia process in CLL. As soon as treatment has finished, lymphocytes will begin to replicate themselves again.

There are also other types of cells that fight infections, including white blood cells and neutrophyls. They migrate to sites of injury and engulf bacteria. The numbers of these are shown in the WBC Differential. Our overall white blood cell count rises significantly during periods of illness or infection but the level drops back subsequently as we fight off the infection. The levels need to be monitored but we can still survive when our white blood cells count is well above the norm. The levels will go down during chemotherapy treatment.

Red blood cells (RBC) and Haemoglobin (HGB)

Red blood cells are generated in the bone marrow. These are the cells that contain haemoglobin. When we breathe in, the air moves amongst millions of tiny porous blood vessels in the lungs where an exchange of gases takes place. Red blood cells in contact with the air absorb oxygen from the air. Haemoglobin is a remarkable protein that combines with oxygen inside red blood cells. When the red blood cells enter the capillaries of the lungs, the haemoglobin takes up oxygen to carry round the body. The oxygen is passed to organs and muscles to enable our bodies to function. Carbon dioxide (the waste product) is then taken back to the lungs and breathed out. Our breathing out also contains some unused oxygen too.

Breathing is a pretty efficient process given that our air has many gases in it, such as oxygen, nitrogen, carbon dioxide and other trace gases. The process is efficient except in extreme circumstances, such as under water, at the top of mountains where the air is thin, and where toxic gases (such as carbon monoxide or sulphur dioxide) are present. However, the efficiency is dependent on our having a plentiful supply of red blood cells and haemoglobin. Red blood cells have a life span of between 90 - 120 days, decaying at a rate of about 1% per day.

A shortage of red blood cells leads to symptoms of anaemia. This can occur during chemotherapy treatment. Normal red blood cells are fairly robust but chemotherapy treatment may create conditions in the blood that can tear these cells apart (haemolysis) or stop our bone marrow producing red blood cells (red blood cell aplasia).

Our bodies need a satisfactory intake of iron in our diet to produce haemoglobin and red blood cells. Like every other ingredient in our diet, it is necessary to maintain a balance. There is a maximum amount of iron that the body can absorb - excess is usually excreted.

We can avoid low levels of haemoglobin most of the time by including iron-rich elements or supplements in our diet. If life were simple, we would just eat more of these foods and achieve a good level of iron for our blood cells. No such luck! Some of the iron-rich foods have drawbacks, which is why we always need to check with a doctor or dietician or qualified herbalist if we change our diet or take health supplements.

If your red blood cell and haemoglobin levels drop very low you may be advised to have a blood transfusion or a series of transfusions, as happened to me (see page 36). **NB. Stop all iron supplements during periods of blood transfusions.** The donated blood transfusion gives you a high intake of iron. Additional iron would cause an excess which might then need to be treated. You may be advised to take a course of treatment involving steroids (see page 37).

Platelets

Platelets are small non-cellular fragments which clot, that is, stick tightly to damaged tissue resulting from an injury. This forms a sticky film over the open cut or wound and gradually hardens into a scab. This closes the wound, preventing further loss of blood and protecting us from infection. The scab allows new skin and tissue to grow underneath in safety. When the cut or wound has healed, the scab of dead cells dries up completely and comes off. The platelets provide the first response to blood clotting, within the body and on broken skin. They have a short life of 8 - 14 days.

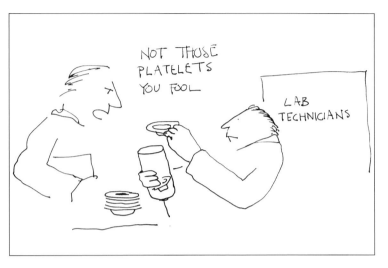

Our platelet levels can go down with CLL and especially during treatment such as chemotherapy. This leaves us very vulnerable to injuries which do not heal quickly and more susceptible to bleeding.

During the early years of the illness, we are likely to recover from most of these injuries and bruises, slowly but satisfactorily. Sometimes, treatment or the illness may reduce the levels of platelets to the point where you need a platelet transfusion (see page 37).

Never look down to test the ground before taking the next step; only he who keeps his eye fixed on the far horizon will find his right road.

Dag Hammarskjold, 1905 – 1961, Swedish statesman and Secretary-General of the United Nations.

Treatments

Chemotherapy

The very word 'chemotherapy' can cause feelings of worry. Our imaginations may begin to work overtime, thinking of worst-case scenarios. However, there have been big advances in medicine and in the treatment of CLL, so in the initial stages of the disease the chemotherapy prescribed (e.g. chlorambucil) may have fairly limited effects on us. Chemotherapy is prescribed to reduce the level of lymphocyte cells and is usually followed by a period of remission.

In the initial stages, the medication is most likely to be taken orally, allowing us to administer and manage our own treatment at home. We may feel the symptoms of CLL somewhat more severely, such as an increase in fatigue, swollen and uncomfortable lymph nodes, anaemia and an increased vulnerability to infection. (See earlier text on how to manage the symptoms.)

These symptoms often lessen during the 6 month period of chemotherapy. We are usually prescribed an additional medication to reduce any sickness arising from taking oral chemotherapy. During the period of chemotherapy, we will be asked to attend for more frequent blood tests so the consultants can monitor the symptoms and effects of the treatment.

Our bodies generally become accustomed to the first type of chemotherapy, so as the years go by it becomes necessary to prescribe other types of chemotherapy, which serve the same purpose but which may have more severe side effects. At this point, there is great variation of response in individual people and this book cannot attempt to advise individual cases, although many of the ways we manage our illness will still apply. For ideas on managing fatigue, swollen lymph nodes, anaemia and infections, see the ideas on pages 9-25.

Occasionally, some of us will develop haemolysis - a reduction in red blood cells and haemoglobin - or red blood cell aplasia where our red blood cell production stops. In these circumstances, we may be advised to have a blood transfusion (see below), but we can manage this too and survive to tell the tale. There are differing forms of treatment that may kick-start the production of red blood cells again and give us another period of remission. Research into CLL is not widespread yet but is being carried out. This is a reason for giving additional blood samples when requested by our consultants. The more the consultants can test, the greater the chances that their research will eventually achieve successful outcomes for us.

Blood Transfusions

If your red blood count and haemoglobin levels go down, this may leave you feeling weak, very tired and breathless after quite ordinary exertion, such as climbing stairs. You may feel your heart pounding and experience cramps more frequently. These are some of the symptoms of anaemia. There may be others indicated by your consultant. In such cases, your doctor may wish to raise your red blood count and haemoglobin levels by means of a blood transfusion.

This is a time-consuming and uncomfortable procedure but will restore your energy. Usually you will be told in advance when to attend (this gives the hospital time to match your blood) and roughly how long the process will last. Each unit of blood may take between 1^1/$_2$ and 2^1/$_2$ hours to absorb, plus preparation time and a little recovery time before and after the procedure. The blood you will be given will match your own, will probably be concentrated or rich in red blood cells and will be irradiated blood. This is blood that has been treated, so that any lymphocytes from the donor will be prevented from reacting to or attacking your own blood cells. **Any further blood transfusions must also be irradiated blood** - you will be given a card to carry with you so that if at any time you need a transfusion for a sudden injury, medical staff will know that you need irradiated blood only.

You may be given the treatment either in the day-room with other patients, or in a room of your own, either of which will allow the nurses to monitor your condition. You will have a comfortable seat or bed with nearby toilet facility. The nurse in charge of your treatment will identify a suitable vein on one of your arms and insert a cannula which will connect, via a tube and valve, to the bag of donor blood. There may be some initial pain or discomfort from this but this usually goes down, leaving you with the simple discomfort of an attachment to a bag looped on an upright walking-trolley. This trolley will allow you to move around with care, visit the toilet, etc. Your condition will be checked regularly - blood pressure, temperature, pulse - to ensure your condition remains stable.

What positive strategies can we use to manage the process?

- Wear comfortable, loose clothing, including socks.

- Take a warm jacket or shawl in case you need it.

- Take some bottled water - there will probably be a drinking water fountain nearby but it will require getting up and down and may be very cold to drink.

- Take some easy to carry, simple food, such as fruit, sponge cake or biscuits. You will be offered a sandwich or something at lunchtime, but it can be helpful to have something extra of your own or something more suited to your dietary preferences.

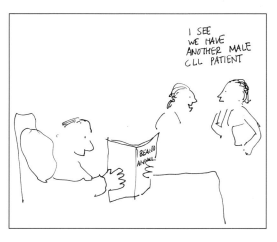

- Take one or two easy-to-read books or magazines to distract you during the procedure.

  At my first transfusion, the nurse laughed at my choice of book - a crime thriller called 'Blood on the Wood'.... ouch!... but it helped pass the time!

- Take a Walkman or personal stereo with tapes or discs of enjoyable music and/or stories.

- If you have friends or family with time to spare, invite one of them to visit you for a while - chatting can make the time pass more quickly. It can help them to feel good about helping you get through the day.

  The wise man does not lay up treasure. The more he gives to others, the more he has for his own.
  Lao-Tze, c.600 BC. Chinese philosopher and founder of Taoism

- Take an elasticated sleeping mask, like those used on airline flights and available in pharmacies and airport general stores. A mask makes it easier to doze off in a very brightly lit room.

- You can monitor your own blood intake by noticing when the unit is almost empty. Nursing staff are usually very observant, but they do have a busy schedule. By notifying the nurse when the unit is nearly empty, you will be able to start the next unit without a long pause in between, or complete the process and go home.

NB. Remember - do not take iron supplements if you are receiving treatment by blood transfusion. The donor blood is rich in iron and this might build up in your system.

Platelet Transfusions

Platelets, made in the bone marrow, have a short life-span of only 8-14 days. If your level of platelets goes too low, it may be necessary to have a transfusion of platelets. In this case, the transfusion will consist of a concentrate of platelet blood cells with many other blood cells removed. The procedure is similar to that of Blood Transfusion above, and the strategies suggested will be the same.

Steroids

Steroids can sometimes be prescribed if your bone marrow stops producing red blood cells. You may be given a bone marrow biopsy to ascertain if this is the case. For some people this is not too painful a process, but for other people it is carried out with a sedative first. Nothing is prescribed without thought and consideration for all your symptoms. Doctors will try a range of chemicals to help you fight the illness.

If you are prescribed steroids, you will be told about the potential positive effects, that is to kick-start your bone marrow into producing red blood cells again and reduce the growth of lymphocyte cells.

Of course, all medication can have side effects and this is true of steroids. Your doctor and pharmacist and the medication leaflet that comes with the steroids will warn you of these. Many of the symptoms will be an aggravation of the symptoms you may already suffer. You may be prescribed medication alongside the steroids, such as antibiotics, to reduce sickness while you are being treated with steroids. And if you are prescribed steroids for any length of time (e.g. 6 months), there is an increasing risk of loss of bone calcium (osteoporosis) for which you will be prescribed a calcium supplement.

- **Increased risk of infection (See also page 13)**

  Treatment with steroids leaves us more exposed and vulnerable to infections. You will need to be very careful during this time to avoid people with known infections, particularly in the winter months when it is more difficult to throw off infections. Make the most of opportunities when you and the family are relatively free of illness, and accept that visits may be further apart during the cold season.

- **Changes in blood pressure (see also page 25)**

  Your blood pressure can become erratic during treatment. Changes as simple as sitting up suddenly or going upstairs can increase your pulse rate and make you feel faint. This is a time for learning: make physical movements a little more slowly to allow you body to adjust. Your doctor/consultant will monitor your blood pressure during this time.

- **Reduction of bone calcium leading to osteoporosis**

  If you are an elderly person, this may be a condition you have already discussed with your GP. However, this is a real possibility when taking steroids for any length of time. In my own case, no-one suggested that I be given a bone density scan when I was first prescribed steroids, with the result that I developed osteoporosis. It was only when I experienced severe back pain that I was given an X-ray, which showed the loss of bone and led to further scans and treatment.

  So, if you are prescribed steroids, insist on a bone density scan to check the condition of your bones. You may be then prescribed with daily calcium tablets (not unpleasant chewy tablets) and possible other medication (such as Residronate) to sustain and/or restore bone calcium.

- **Poor sleep patterns (see also page 19)**

  The hospital pharmacist can give you very good advice about combating side effects. For example, the pharmacist advised me to take the steroid tablets in the morning with food, as taking them in the evening can make sleep less easy.

  - **Increased susceptibility to bruising (see page 18)**
  - **Fluid retention: e.g. giving swollen ankles, facial swelling (see page 22)**
  - **Weight gain (see page 22)**
  - **Stomach upsets and diarrhoea (see page 23)**

The Pharmacy and Medication

If you are prescribed medication for CLL, such as chemotherapy by oral tablets, you will normally be directed to the hospital pharmacy for oncology prescriptions. It is likely that you will be given the prescription following your blood test and consultation. Depending on the way the hospital trust organises the pharmaceutical staff, you may have to wait some time for the prescribed medication. I have never waited much less than 30 minutes, occasionally over an hour and once waited 3 hours. This waiting, on top of the time already spent in the hospital, can cause distress.

Do bear in mind that it is not the fault of the pharmacists. They are as concerned as we are to fill the prescriptions quickly, but they have limited staff. We can minimise the distress such waiting around can cause:

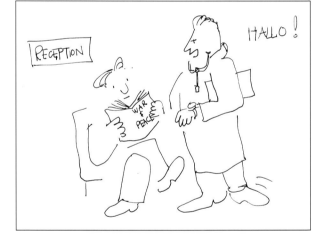

- Resign yourself in advance to a longish wait.

- Take a good book to read or earphones to listen to music.

- Go away and return later.

- Have a coffee and chat with your friend or family.

If the wait is unnecessarily long (more than an hour), let the Hospital Site Manager or Hospital Trust know. Inflicting distress on patients is not going to help our recovery and Hospital Managers should look for ways to avoid this.

Information

The pharmacist will explain the directions for taking the medication. You may not have had enough time to address any questions with your consultant, or you may need reassurance that you have understood the instructions. The pharmacist is the person to check the doctor's recommendations and ask questions about:

- dosage

- frequency of taking the medication

- time of day

- where to store the medication

- possible side effects and how to manage these

- dietary considerations

- what you might do if you feel sick or not well enough to eat (many prescriptions suggest taking medication with food)

- what you might do if you have difficulty swallowing the medication

- whether you are allowed to drink alcohol during this treatment, and how much

- whether other medication you are taking or health foods will interfere with it

    In my case I was unwittingly taking a counter-productive health supplement during treatment, and only found out by having a discussion with the pharmacist.

What strategies can we use for storing and taking medication?

It is often recommended that prescribed medications are kept at a cool temperature, taken with or just after food, or taken with fluids. Try to establish a routine with your medication that suits you and your life schedule, such as:

- Store them in a cool part of the refrigerator, unless otherwise recommended.

- Store them near your milk so that you are always reminded to take them out when you have your breakfast (if this time is recommended).

- Most medication is to be taken with or just after a meal. If possible, try taking them at breakfast time. That way, the one-a-day tablets won't have to be carried around with you during the day or evening. Make the meal an enjoyable one, something to look forward to, so that the medication becomes incidental to it.

- Drink plenty of fluids with your medication.

- Choose enjoyable fluids to drink with your medication, such as orange juice, tea, herbal tea, sparkling mineral water, apple juice, etc. (not alcohol).

- Buy a nice little cool bag to carry around any tablets you do have to take more than once a day. This is also useful to carry medication when visiting family or on holiday.

NB. Return any old or unused medicines to the pharmacy for safe disposal.

Support for People with CLL

There are unexpected financial aspects when we are diagnosed with CLL. For example, normal travel insurance will not cover those of us with an existing condition such as CLL, and we have to pay an additional cost for medical insurance, which may be as expensive as the holiday itself. One hidden cost which can mount up over the months and years is the cost of transport, whether to and from the hospital or anywhere else.

For 8 years I traipsed backwards and forward to the hospital using public transport - walking + 2 train changes each way. Then that became too difficult to manage. In one year, I have spent over £500 in parking fees just visiting the hospital. I now have an Attendance Allowance. If anyone had advised me sooner, I would not have had to face such costs. It is important to think about such costs and take steps to get the best financial support for yourself, and apply for any benefits sooner rather than later.

CLL may be expensive in ways that we never expect, such as extra child care, the cost of prescriptions or a special diet. But there is help available if we are struggling to cope with the costs of CLL. This section isn't a complete guide, but it is an attempt to list some of the main types of support that may be needed.

Disability Living Allowance or Attendance Allowance

Disability Living Allowance is for people under 65; Attendance Allowance is for people over 65. Both of them are for people who need help looking after themselves. For example, if you need help getting out of bed, washing, dressing, using the toilet or cooking, then it's quite likely that you will be entitled to one of these allowances. If you do receive one of these allowances then you might find that you are entitled to other kinds of support as well.

Income Support or Pension Credit

These are benefits that can top-up your income, if you are working, or your pension if you are old enough to receive a pension. The amount that you get will depend on how much income and savings you have. Although they are means-tested, quite a lot of people are entitled to this extra support. If you receive Income Support then you automatically become entitled to other kinds of support, like free prescriptions. If you are well enough to keep on working when you have CLL, then an additional benefit is called the **Disabled Persons' Tax Credit.** This is another benefit that helps to top-up your income. If you become too ill to work then you may be able to get **Incapacity Benefit.** You may be able to claim this even if you are self-employed or unemployed.

Transport

In the first stages of the illness, you may only be visiting the hospital for blood tests and checks once every 3 months. If the hospital is reasonably near and you are still feeling strong and mobile, this may not involve you in a great expense. You might be travelling by public transport, so parking fees may not be a problem. You may be able to claim a refund of your travel costs to the hospital. Some charitable organisations have volunteer drivers who can give people lifts to hospitals. Your local library should have details.

If your condition deteriorates, public transport may no longer be a comfortable option and you may be forced to rely on other means of transport. You can check if you can be collected, delivered and returned from the hospital by the ambulance service. This would be free of charge but be warned . . . waiting times can be very long at either end of the visit!

You may need to travel by taxi. This can be expensive if your visits are frequent. You may find it easier to travel to the hospital (and elsewhere) by car, in which case you will almost undoubtedly will incur parking fees. Travelling by car can give us the confidence to visit the hospital in greater comfort and be more mobile the rest of the time as we become less able to use public transport. You may qualify for a Disabled Person's Badge for your car. A Disabled Person's Badge allows us to park the car nearer to the hospital or shops etc. and reduces the distances we have to walk.

Many parking places will be either designated Disabled, or free of charge all day (Parking Bays), or for up to 3 hours (e.g. Single Yellow Lines). However some councils continue to charge Disabled Drivers, so you must always check the information if you are given a Disabled Person's Badge. It is really a great blessing and removes a great deal of stress when you are moving around. In London, if you have a Disabled Person's Badge, you will also qualify for free passage through the Congestion Charge Zone. You will be able to nominate your own car and/or the car in which you travel regularly as a passenger. It is very helpful. Contact **Transport for London** for details.

There are special rates for bus and rail travel for people with disabilities. For example, a Disabled Person's Railcard will give you a third off the cost of most journeys by train. Check at your local bus or train station for details.

Health costs

As most of us with CLL are usually older, our prescriptions may already be free of charge. If not, do check that you are not incurring costs unnecessarily. You may be entitled to:

- free prescriptions
- free NHS dental treatment
- free NHS sight tests and eye treatment
- subsidised glasses or contact lenses

- free NHS wigs and fabric supports
- special equipment or aids, such as a raised toilet seat

If you are claiming Income Support or Disabled Persons' Tax Credit then you should get these automatically. If you aren't claiming one of these benefits, then you might still be entitled to free prescriptions if your income is low enough.

Other state benefits

If you are on a low income or receiving Income support then there are other benefits that you may be able to claim. **Housing Benefit** and **Council Tax Benefit** will help with your rent or accommodation costs, including things like mortgage interest payments and service charges. You may be able to get help to adapt your home - e.g. by putting in a ramp, stairlift or central heating. You may be able to get a key for access to public toilets for disabled people. **Social Fund** grants may cover things like heating costs, replacing a washing machine or funeral costs.

Travel insurance

Travel insurance costs will rocket now you have CLL. Apart from the usual cover for cancellations, lost luggage, etc., travel companies and insurance agencies will insist on medical cover. The cost of medical insurance when you travel abroad may be particularly expensive.

> *It is tempting to do without additional medical cover, as those of us with CLL during remission periods may feel very well. However, it is a mistake not to have appropriate cover - my own bitter experience in cancelling just 2 holidays in 8 years has cost me very dear!*

However, some companies offer more favourable packages, such as that recommended by CancerBACUP. Do some research to find out the best deal - after all, for many years we may be either in remission or not exhibiting extreme symptoms that will need medical attention during the times when we are away on holiday. One possible place to start is Medici Travel Insurance, Tel. 0845 8800 168, www.medicitravel.com

How to apply for support

This can be quite complicated. State benefits are handled by several different agencies. The main ones are:

- Benefits Agency, 0800 882200 or www.dss.gov.uk
- Jobcentre Plus, the agency for benefits for people of working age, www.jobcentreplus.gov.uk
- Pension Service, the agency for benefits for people of pensionable age, www.thepensionservice.gov.uk
- Disability and Carers Service, the agency for benefits for disabled people and their carers, www.dwp.gov.uk

  (These contact details may change)

The best place to start is to contact your local social services office (it should be listed in the telephone book) and request to see a social worker. The social worker should be able to advise you on what benefits you can claim and how to claim them.

Your local council may have a Welfare Rights unit, where someone will be able to give you advice. Some of the benefits (e.g. Housing Benefit) come from your local council.

Your GP should be able to point you in the right direction if you have any difficulty in contacting the right person to help you. Some of the benefits (e.g. the Disabled Person's Badge for your car) require your GP's support.

Your local Citizen's Advice Bureau will also be able to give you advice about what you are entitled to and help with filling in the claim forms. Your local library may have other useful information.

There are lots of charitable organisations that provide information and advice. Some of the most important ones are listed later. Some of these organisations (e.g. Macmillan Cancer Support) also provide direct financial and medical support.

Investments and Annuities

Many of us who contract CLL are approaching retirement or have reached that age. It may be that you have a sum of money from a pension fund that you could invest in an annuity. You can make more of this sum by buying an annuity based on a shortened life expectancy - one of the few benefits of having CLL! The life insurance company would approach your GP and/or consultant for confirmation of the projected life expectancy, but it is worth it as an annuity of this kind can give a much higher return per month.

Do inform your GP and consultant as these people can differ on your projected life span.

> My own GP contradicted my consultant by giving me a much longer life span than the consultant did. The company accepted my GP's estimation (although she had less experience) and reduced their offer accordingly. This has cost me a great deal of money over the last 5 years.

Consult your own financial adviser, if you have one, or try a range of life insurance companies.

Recent Advances in Research and Treatment in Chronic Lymphocytic Leukaemia

Dr. A.G. Prentice, Consultant Haematologist

Royal Free Hampstead NHS Trust, London

In the past two decades, scientists and clinicians have begun to make real progress in defining how this disease develops and in how to treat it. It is becoming clearer that this is not just one disease but a spectrum of disorders, which may look the same in a blood count or film at any one time, but which can behave very differently. Some patients have CLL which develops very slowly and may never need any treatment, while others have a more aggressive disease which may need treatment as soon as the diagnosis is made. The simplest way to distinguish patients at these two ends of the spectrum is to look at how quickly the lymphocyte count doubles. If this takes less than 6 months then treatment will be needed soon, but if it takes longer than a year, treatment may be delayed without harm.

Some patients find it difficult to accept that treatment need not be given simply because the white cell count is high. The speed of increase is much more important. Fast doubling times are associated more with disease which doctors and patients can feel in enlarged lymph glands and the spleen. They are also seen with the progressive anaemia and thrombocytopenia (low blood platelets needed to prevent bleeding and bruising) which reflect replacement of the bone marrow by CLL cells.

Two main systems of staging of patients with CLL are used by doctors: the Binet and the Rai systems, which are very similar. They may sound very technical but they simply reflect degrees of aggressiveness of the disease and act as a guide to the need for treatment. These systems can be supported by further evidence of the extent and state of the disease using CT scanning (which shows lymph node enlargement where we cannot feel it) and a bone marrow biopsy (which shows how much disease is infiltrating the bone marrow and the pattern of infiltration).

Not all patients need these tests at the outset, particularly if they have little or no enlargement of lymph glands which can be felt, if they have low CLL cell counts in the blood, if they have no anaemia or other evidence of failure of normal bone marrow production, and if their CLL counts are stable or rising only very slowly. Minimal investigation means less distress for patients who will not benefit from it or who do not need immediate treatment.

We can get more useful information about the likely future behaviour of the disease in individuals from recent advances in sophisticated blood tests. These look as if they can separate patients whose disease will progress rapidly from those whose disease may never need to be treated. Not all of these tests tell us who will benefit from treatment, or which type of treatment we should use, but some do.

There are three main types of test. The first is to look in detail at the chromosomes within the CLL cells (cytogenetics). There we can see that some CLL families (clones) have lost or mutated key genes which control either the repair of DNA or are able to suppress the development of tumours. Depending on which gene is affected, we can predict which patients are likely to progress more rapidly and which are likely to be resistant to chemotherapy.

For example, deletion or mutation of a part of chromosome 17 leads to failure to produce a protein called p53, which is responsible both for DNA repair and for a pathway through which drugs can kill tumour cells. If we detect this abnormality, we can predict which kind of treatment we need to use to gain some control over the CLL.

We can also detect the presence of the p53 molecule within the cell by other molecular techniques. Molecular techniques can be used to determine whether receptors on the surface of the cell have been mutated, and the degree of mutation can predict how aggressively the disease will behave. The state of these receptors might determine how the CLL cell responds to signals from other types of cells in its surroundings in lymph nodes and bone marrow. These responses could decide how aggressive the disease will become.

In addition, we can study the surface of the CLL cell using a technique called flow cytometry. This enables us to detect the expression of other surface receptors or markers of the disease. These may also predict its behaviour, but not necessarily how it will respond to different forms of treatment. Two types of receptor have been studied intensively, CD38 and ZAP70. There is much discussion about which is the more powerful predictor of progression and which method is the most reliable for their detection.

Finding this new information about how CLL 'works' has encouraged the development of new types of treatment. Treatment with drugs was largely confined to simple oral chlorambucil until recently. It is becoming clearer that we can get better and longer lasting responses to treatment if we use combinations of drugs, such as fludarabine and cyclophosphamide. These combinations presumably weaken the CLL cells' resistance to drug-induced death by attacking them through more than one pathway.

The addition of antibodies to drugs may enhance their effect by attacking the cell through yet another pathway. We have two antibodies which work in this way. One is anti-CD20 (rituximab) and the other anti-CD56 (alemtuzumab), which attack different receptors and trigger cell death pathways. They are very expensive and the NHS is reluctant to fund their use, at least not in patients who have not yet had another more conventional drug treatment, such as chlorambucil. Anti-CD56 has the added advantage of by-passing the mutated or missing p53 obstacle which makes CLL cells resistant to drug-induced death. There will be other antibody treatments soon and the next one (anti-CD23) is entering trials in N. America and Europe now.

The latest development has been in stem cell transplantation. We are now able to transplant patients with CLL with stem cells from matched donors (usually related) when they are resistant to chemotherapy. It is becoming clearer that this is best done earlier in the course of the disease, rather than later when patients have been repeatedly harmed by cumulative side effects of drugs. So our ability to predict aggressiveness and resistance to chemotherapy in this disease becomes even more important, allowing us to plan transplants earlier in the course of the disease in patients who are fitter and less harmed by prior drug therapy. Results of these transplants are at an early stage, and this procedure is not undertaken lightly.

Much progress has been made in the increasing understanding of the biology of CLL, and this is now beginning to show rewards in a greater breadth of treatment options. There remains the need for careful and skilful selection of patients for these specific therapies and for much more research.

Recipes and Diet

Minerals and Vitamins

These not only contribute to our general health but act as antioxidants which help to prevent heart disease and cancer. However, too much of anything can be just as bad as too little. Moderation and a balanced diet is essential.

Buy fresh fruit and vegetables and store them in cool conditions. When cooking, cook just before serving to prevent loss of the important vitamins and minerals. Wash or scrub just before cooking, chop as little as necessary to reduce the amount of cut surface. Use the least water for boiling or try to steam or microwave to avoid leaching the goodness.

Calcium (for bones & teeth) is found in milk, cheese, eggs, canned fish, shellfish, beans, green and root vegetables, enriched white flour and breads.

NB. Note that some foods act as calcium 'thieves', inhibiting the body's ability to absorb calcium. So don't consume too many of the following: caffeine, animal protein, salt, phosphates or alcohol.

Iron (for blood & haemoglobin) is found in wholegrain cereals and breads, lean meat, fish, pulses, leafy green vegetables and potatoes, prunes and other dried fruits, parsley.

Vitamin A (for good skin, glands & bones) is found in milk, cheese, butter, some margarines, eggs, carrots, spinach and other green vegetables, tomatoes, watercress, blueberries and blackberries, dried apricots and other 'orange' fruit and veg. such as squash, sweet potatoes, prunes, avocados, fish oils.

Vitamin B (supports the nervous system) is found in baker's yeast, wholegrain cereals, lean meat, ham and bacon, milk and cheese, fruit, nuts.

Vitamin C (helps our resistance to infection) is found in blackberries and blueberries, citrus fruits and juices, kiwi fruit, fresh vegetables (not overcooked).

Vitamin D (assists the take up of calcium for our bones) is found in fish oils, egg yolk, butter, some margarines, and made with sunlight on the skin.

Vitamin E is found in vegetable oils especially corn, soya bean, olive, canola and sunflower oils and margarines, wholegrain foods, nuts and seeds.

Vitamin K (helps blood to clot) is found in spinach, lettuce, brassicas (e.g. cabbage, broccoli), cereals, dairy products and eggs.

Taking this information into account, a healthy daily diet for CLL sufferers might look something like this.

● Wholegrain cereal and bread.

● 5 portions of fresh or dried fruit and vegetables - cooked just soft enough to eat (al dente), using vegetable oils and margarines (check the ingredients on the packet).

If you aim for a 'rainbow' of fruit, vegetables and juices, you will be fairly sure of getting the best range of vitamins and minerals.

red: beetroot, strawberries, raspberries, tomatoes

orange: oranges, mangoes, peaches, apricots, carrots, sweet potatoes, lentils

green: cabbage, broccoli, runner beans, salads, kiwi fruit, apples, pears, avocados

blue-purple: blueberries, blackberries, cranberries, plums, prunes

white: potatoes, turnips, leeks, onions

● Select 1-2 daily portions from dairy or soya milk, cheese (especially cottage cheese), lean meat, fish (including oily fish such as sardines, salmon and kippers), soya products (such as tofu), pulses (such as lentils and beans), eggs.

● Season with a range of herbs and spices, especially chives, parsley

Occasionally each week: Nuts and seeds (if not allergic to these)

Most of us don't usually achieve the 'perfect diet', but that doesn't matter. Do the best you can and make sure you give yourself treats from time to time!

Suggestions for Healthy Recipes

I have tried to give quantities in metric and imperial measurements, as well as 'spoon-sized' measures, so you can use whichever one you feel most comfortable with.

In most cases you don't have to use the exact quantities given in the recipe. Usually you can use a bit more or less, or substitute ingredients with whatever you happen to have available. Experiment and see what works for you.

Home-made Muesli

Make in quantity and keep in an airtight box or self-seal plastic bag

50g / 2 tbsp rolled oats
25g / 1tbsp quinoa (optional, use if available)
50g / 2 tbsp raisins or sultanas
50g / 2 tbsp chopped, soft dried apricots
25g / 1 tbsp dried apple slices (optional, use if available)
50g / 2 tbsp chopped hazelnuts or walnuts (optional)

Combine the ingredients and add soya milk, low fat milk or yoghurt and top with fresh fruit such as slices of banana, berries or grapes.

Fruity Rutin (a great breakfast starter or dessert at any time)

1 large orange
1 or 2 other fruits as available - apple, kiwi fruit, grapes, banana

PREPARATION

Use a potato peeler or a sharp knife to peel the zest only from the orange, keeping most or some of the pith on the orange. Cut into pieces (keep the zest for adding to a drink or dessert). Cut up the other fruits into bite-sized chunks and mix together.

Eat plain for breakfast, add to your cereals or add non-dairy ice-cream or soya yogurt for a tasty dessert.

This can be prepared the evening before, covered with clingfilm and kept in the fridge.

Watercress and Rocket Salad (2-3 servings)

Half a bunch watercress
1 bunch rocket
1 bunch basil
1 bunch asparagus
1-2 peaches or nectarines
Juice of 1 lemon or lime
2-3 tbsps olive oil
2 tbsps pine nuts
Crushed garlic and pepper to taste

PREPARATION

Wash watercress, rocket and basil. Dry thoroughly, removing unwanted stems or leaves and tear into bite-sized pieces. Arrange in a salad bowl. Cut off woody ends of the asparagus and cut each spear in half. Steam (8 - 12 minutes) or microwave until just tender. Remove skin and stones from the peaches and dice the flesh. Add to the salad bowl with the asparagus and pine nuts.

Just before serving, mix the remaining ingredients together and pour over the salad.

This makes a tasty lunch meal with a hot wholemeal pitta bread.

If just one serving is required, put half the salad into a bowl before pouring the dressing over, cover with clingfilm and keep in the fridge until the following day.

Quick lentil soup (serves 4)

2 onions, chopped
4-6 carrots, cleaned and grated
2-4 turnips, cleaned and grated (optional)
8-10 medium size mushrooms, cleaned and chopped (optional)
100g / 4 tbsp red lentils
2 tbsp grated root ginger or 1 tsp dried ginger
2 pints / 1 litre low salt chicken or vegetable stock
2 cloves garlic, crushed or chopped
4 tbsp olive oil or vegetable oil
Salt and pepper to taste, chopped chives if available

PREPARATION

Fry the onion, garlic and ginger in the olive oil for 3-5 mins until the onion is golden brown. Add the turnips and other chopped vegetables together with the stock. Bring to the boil and simmer gently for 15-20 mins or until the lentils are soft.

Serve with chopped chives or parsley on top, and warmed fresh brown bread.

A pressure cooker can be a great investment - everything not only cooks quickly (5 minutes for the above) but retains almost all the vitamins and minerals in the food.

Leek and potato soup (serves 4)

1 large onion, chopped
2-3 leeks, washed thoroughly and chopped into slices
2-3 medium sized potatoes, peeled and cut into small pieces
1-2 cloves garlic, crushed or chopped
1 tbsp grated root ginger or 1/2 tsp dried ginger
2 pints low salt chicken or vegetable stock
2-3 tbsp olive oil or vegetable oil
Salt and pepper to taste, herbs to garnish

PREPARATION

Fry the onion, garlic, leeks and ginger in the olive oil for 3-5 mins. Add the stock and remaining ingredients and bring to the boil. Simmer gently for approx. 20 mins or until the potatoes are soft and crumbly. Serve with chopped chives or parsley and wholemeal bread. Add lightly-fried pieces of bacon to make the soup into a full meal.

Healthy Sandwiches

As a general rule:

- Use wholemeal bread.

- Use a low fat spread or as little butter or margarine as possible.

- Avoid mayonnaise unless low fat.

- Avoid salty extras such as pickles and chutneys.

Possible fillings:

- Cottage or ricotta cheese + salad, such as cucumber, chives, lettuce, tomatoes

- Low fat or soy cheese + grated apple & grated carrot, lettuce, chopped celery & nuts

- Slices of cooked chicken or turkey + fresh salad

- Tuna or salmon + drizzle of lemon juice & lettuce

- Avocado & soft tofu spread (see below)

- Mashed banana, nuts & raisins & honey

Add a few chopped fresh herbs to any of the above instead of salt, e.g. chopped chives, a little parsley. Sandwich fillings can also be used to turn a baked potato into a main dish (see below).

Avocado & soft tofu filling

I large ripe avocado
Juice of 1/2 lemon
100 g soft tofu
Pinch of black pepper
Pinch of paprika
1 small clove garlic (optional)
A little grated carrot

PREPARATION

Peel and stone the avocado. Use a blender or mash all the ingredients together until smooth. Spread on the bread and top with grated carrot.

Can be used also as a lunchtime or party dip with pieces of wholemeal pitta bread, toast, breadsticks and celery, carrot strips and spring onions.

Stir-fried tofu and broccoli (2 large or 4 smaller servings)

200 g fresh tofu, chopped into small cubes (tofu can be frozen on the day of purchase - it changes texture a little but this can be tasty too)
400g broccoli, chopped into florets
4-5 spring onions, or 3 shallots or 1 small onion, chopped
1 tablespoon olive or sunflower oil
1 clove garlic, chopped or crushed
1 tbsp root ginger, grated
2 carrots, cut into thin strips
100g bean sprouts, washed
50g noodles, fast-cook if possible
1-2 tablespoons cornflour or plain flour
2 tablespoons cold water
1 pint vegetable stock

Marinade:
1/2 pint vegetable stock
1 tablespoon low salt soy sauce
2 tablespoons Hoi Sin Sauce
1 tablespoon dry sherry (optional)

PREPARATION

Combine the ingredients for the marinade. Chop the tofu into small cubes and stir into the marinade. Leave, if possible, for 2-3 hours, stirring regularly to coat the tofu on all sides. (The recipe will still work if you don't have time to marinade the tofu in advance - use as a sauce to add to the pan with the tofu.)

Heat the oil in a deep saucepan or wok. Fry the spring onions and garlic for 2-3 minutes. Add the tofu and marinade sauce and the carrot strips. Fry for a further 3-4 minutes, stirring frequently. If the stir-fry starts to dry out - add a little more water or stock.

Meanwhile cook the noodles in boiling water, according to the instructions on the packet (approx. 3-4 minutes). Drain and keep warm in the pan until needed.

Mix the flour with the cold water and set aside until needed later.

Add the broccoli to the tofu mixture and cook for another 5-8 minutes. Don't overcook at this stage - keep testing the vegetables so they are just tender. Stir in the beansprouts and cook for 2 more minutes. Stir in the cooked noodles and the flour mixture a little at a time until the stir-fry thickens (approx.1-2 minutes).

Other vegetables work in this dish as well as or instead of the broccoli e.g. Pak choy, courgettes, string beans, mange-touts, etc., but bear in mind cooking times may vary. You don't need anything else to serve with this dish but wholemeal or pitta bread helps to mop up some of the juices!

Baked potato

Scrub clean a large potato, spike with a skewer and/or prick the skin with a fork. Cook in a moderate oven (gas mark 5,190°C) for approx. 1 hour until a skewer or sharp knife goes into the centre quite easily. Cut in half and allow to cool a little. Serve with one of the sandwich fillings above or home made coleslaw.

Potatoes are a good source of fibre with the same number of calories as an apple. The vitamins and minerals are just under the skin so we need to eat them either washed or very thinly peeled, and cooked just before eating. If boiling, use just enough water to cover the potatoes and re-use the boiled water for stock or to cook rice or pasta. Microwaving potatoes is quicker but makes the skin go soggy.

Home made Coleslaw

225g / 8 oz red or green or white cabbage, shredded
225g / 8 oz carrots, in thin strips
50g / 2 oz beansprouts or alfalfa sprouts, washed (add just before use if you have them)
9 mls / 6 tsp low fat mayonnaise

PREPARATION

Clean and chop the vegetables into thin narrow strips. Mix together and add just enough mayonnaise to coat the vegetables.

Use what you need and keep the rest in an airtight container in the fridge. It will comfortably last 3-4 days.

You can ring the changes by adding 2-3 celery sticks (chopped), or 25g / 1 oz pine nuts or pumpkin seeds, or 50-75g / 2-3 oz chopped dried apricots.

Potato and Leek Gratin (serves 4-6)

2 leeks, chopped
2 onions, chopped
4 tbsp olive oil
2 large potatoes, chopped into bite-sized pieces.
100 g chopped mushrooms (optional)
300 g fresh tofu
50 g cheddar cheese, grated
3-4 tbsp chopped parsley
3-4 tbsp chopped chives
2 tbsp tamari soy sauce
150 ml soya milk
1 tsp ground black pepper

PREPARATION

Boil the potatoes until just tender. Put into an oven dish. Fry the leeks, onions and mushrooms in half of the oil until tender and add to the potatoes. Whisk the tofu with the remaining ingredients in a blender or food processor. Pour the mixture over the vegetables. Sprinkle the grated cheese over the top. Bake at gas mark 4 / 1800C for 25 mins until the surface is browning.

Spinach and hazelnut lasagne (2 servings)

225g / 8 oz fresh or frozen spinach
100g / 4 oz hazelnuts or pine nuts or other chopped nuts
350g / 12-14 oz fresh or dried lasagne
1 large (12-14 oz) tin of chopped tomatoes or approx. 400g of your own tomato sauce, page 57
1 large or 2 medium onions, chopped
2 tbsp vegetable oil
100g / 4 oz grated cheddar or parmesan cheese
Salt and pepper to taste
Choose 1 tsp of one or more herbs/spices from: dried oregano, dried marjoram, dried thyme or ground nutmeg

White sauce:
75-80g / 3 oz low fat margarine (or use butter if you are trying to restore weight)

50g / 2 oz/ 2 tbsp wholewheat or plain flour
450 ml / 3/4 pint soya milk or dairy milk
Pinch salt

PREPARATION

White sauce: Melt the margarine or butter gently in a saucepan. Stir in the flour and salt. Add the milk little by little and use a whisk to make a smooth mixture. Bring back gently to the boil, stirring all the time. Watch as the sauce thickens - you need a sauce that is like a thick cream rather than porridge. If the sauce seems to be getting too thick, stir in a little more milk or water. Sprinkle a little milk or water over the surface (to prevent a skin forming whilst you prepare the rest), cap with a lid then put to one side.

Defrost the spinach (if frozen) according to instructions on the packet. With fresh spinach, wash well, shake off any residual water and cook in a saucepan over minimal heat, stirring occasionally, until the spinach has become soft. Stir in the hazelnuts and herbs.

Chop the onions and fry them in oil until nearly transparent, then stir in the chopped tomatoes.

Follow instructions regarding cooking the lasagne on the packet. Create layers between the lasagne as follows: white sauce / lasagne / onions + tomatoes / white sauce / lasagne / spinach + nuts / white sauce / lasagne / white sauce (top with cheese if desired).

Cook in a moderate oven, gas mark 4, 180°C for 35-45 minutes. If necessary, grill for 1-3 minutes to brown the surface before serving.

Home made Tomato Sauce (for pasta, pizza and other dishes)

$1^1/_2$ kg fresh tomatoes (fresh is best but you could use a tin of chopped tomatoes if short of time or tomatoes)
2 tablespoons olive oil
1 large onion or 3 shallots, chopped small
2 cloves of garlic, crushed
2 teaspoons sugar
Salt and pepper to taste
Fresh basil for use on the day

PREPARATION

Stand the tomatoes in boiling water for 1 minute. Drain, cool, skin and chop into small pieces. Fry the garlic and onion in the olive oil for about 5 minutes, then stir in the tomatoes and bring to the boil. Simmer gently, stirring regularly for about 25 - 30 minutes until the sauce thickens. Add salt and pepper to taste. Use fresh, or freeze in bags or in ice-cube trays. Use for spaghetti, lasagne, pizza toppings, casseroles, etc.

Salmon fish cakes (4 servings)

225g / 8 oz fresh or tinned salmon
A little milk if using fresh salmon
1 medium onion or 2 shallots
450g / 1 lb sweet potatoes or ordinary potatoes
2-3 tablespoons olive oil
1 egg, beaten
1 tbsp chopped parsley
Salt and pepper to taste

To serve: fresh chopped coriander, parsley or chives / slices of lemon or tomato sauce

PREPARATION

Peel, chop and boil the potatoes for about 20 mins until tender enough for mashing.

Poach the pieces of fresh salmon in enough milk to cover them in either the oven or a saucepan (if using a tin of salmon, drain well and flake the fish).

Fry the chopped onion until golden and add to the mashed potato and flaked, cooked salmon. Add beaten egg, parsley, salt and pepper to taste. Mould into fish cakes approx. 7 cm (3 inches) in diameter.

Heat the olive oil in a frying pan and cook the fish cakes gently on each side until light brown.

Serve with chopped herbs and lemon, with wholemeal rolls and a salad or low-fat oven chips and frozen peas or other vegetable.

The salmon fish cakes can be kept in the refrigerator at this stage for cooking later or wrapped in kitchen foil and frozen for another day.

Roasted butternut squash and rocket risotto (serves 4)

1 butternut squash, peeled, de-seeded and cut into bite-sized chunks
1 tbsp olive oil
Ground black pepper
Risotto:
12 oz / 330g risotto rice
1 garlic clove, crushed
2 oz / 50g butter
1 tbsp olive oil
1 litre hot vegetable stock
3 tbsp sherry
1 tsp tomato puree
1 bay leaf
2 oz / 50g Parmesan cheese, grated
1 tbsp pine nuts
4 oz / 100g rocket

PREPARATION

Roast the squash in the olive oil, with black pepper sprinkled on top in a hot oven (220°C / gas mark 7) for approx. 30 minutes until tender, turning the pieces halfway through. Heat the butter and oil in a non-stick frying pan. Stir in the rice and garlic and cook for 3-4 mins until the rice becomes transparent. Add some of the stock and sherry, tomato puree and bay leaf. Gradually add the remaining stock as it is absorbed by the rice. Keep stirring gently until the rice is cooked (approx. 15-20 mins). Remove the bay leaf.

Add the parmesan and rocket. Serve the risotto with the roasted squash and pine nuts on top.

Smoothies for juicing or food processing

Use a blender, food processor or juicer to create satisfying and healthy drinks for breakfast, lunch or healthy snacks. Make fresh each time.

Banana
1 banana
1 cup soya milk
1 teaspoon chopped walnuts or hazelnuts
1/2 teaspoon vanilla essence

Strawberry / raspberry / blueberry / blackberry Smoothies
10-12 strawberries (depending on the size) or raspberries, blueberries, blackberries
(If the berries are frozen, allow time for them to defrost or use frozen for an iced drink)
1 tablespoon low fat vanilla ice cream or plain yogurt
3/4 cups soya milk
25g / 1 tbsp almond slivers for serving

Carrot and celery pick-me-up (for a juicer machine)
1-2 carrots (peeled and chopped)
2 sticks celery, chopped
Optional extras: a small cooked beetroot, 1-2 spring onions, a handful of beansprouts, a garlic clove, 8-10 stalks of chives

Apple smoothie
1 eating apple, peeled and chopped
1 pear, peeled and chopped
Another skinned, stoned, chopped fruit (e.g. Kiwi fruit/plum/peach/ apricot)

Potato and mushroom curry (serves 4-6)

4 tbsp sunflower oil
1 tsp dried cinnamon or 1 cinnamon stick
2 bay leaves
2 tsp cumin seeds
2 medium onions, chopped into small pieces
2 tbsp finely grated fresh root ginger
6 garlic cloves, crushed
1 tsp tomato puree
4 chopped tomatoes or 1 small tin chopped tomatoes
2 tsp turmeric
2 tsp ground cumin
2 tsp ground coriander
4 medium potatoes, cut into bite-sized pieces
350 g washed small button mushrooms or a mixture of mushrooms (e.g. including shitake and other mushrooms), washed, peeled and chopped
300 ml / half-pint water
2 tbsp tamari

PREPARATION

Fry the cinnamon, bay leaves and cumin seeds in the oil in a deep frying pan or wok for 2-3 mins. Add the onions, ginger, garlic, tomato puree and chopped tomatoes and stir-fry for a few more minutes. Then reduce the heat, cover and cook for a further 10 minutes.

Add the turmeric, ground cumin and coriander and stir well for 2-3 minutes. Add the potatoes and mushrooms, stirring well. Pour in the water and tamari, stir well, cover and cook gently for about 20 - 30 minutes, stirring occasionally until the potatoes are soft.

Serve with rice or warmed pitta or nan bread and a slice of lemon.

Apple and blackberry crumble (serves 4)

3 large cooking apples
1 punnet of blackberries (or blueberries) or 100g berries.
100g/ 4 oz/ 4 tbsp sugar or honey / syrup
2 tsp water

Crumble:
100g / 4 oz / 4 tbsp self-raising flour
50g / 2 oz / 2 tbsp rolled oats (including oats makes it more healthy)
75- 80g / 3 oz low fat margarine
1/2 tbsp allspice or nutmeg
Pinch of salt

PREPARATION

Place the flour in a large bowl and rub in the margarine until the mixture is the consistency of breadcrumbs. Stir in the oats, sugar, salt and spice. Set aside.

Peel and slice the apples and place in a heatproof dish with the water. Spread the blackberries and sugar over the top. Cover with the crumble and cook in a moderate oven (gas mark 5/ 190°C) for about 20-30 mins and the crumble is gently browning. Serve with soya or low fat dairy ice cream.

Make double quantities of the crumble if you can and keep in an airtight plastic container in the fridge for 2-3 weeks. If you leave out the sugar, the mixture makes a good pastry mix for a blackberry and apple pie, bound together with very little water and rolled out on a floured board.

Quick Pancakes (serves 4)

100g / 4-5 tbsp self-raising flour
1 egg
Approx. half a cupful low fat diary milk (soya milk is a bit heavy for this)
Approx. half a cupful water
Pinch of salt
Vegetable oil (sunflower or other)
Low fat butter spread to taste
Sugar, honey or maple syrup to taste
Lemon juice to taste
NB. Non-stick pans may be your only option although they do not give the results that a plain metal frying pan produce.

PREPARATION

Near the cooking area, prepare plates, the butter spread, sugar or honey and lemon juice. Once you are cooking the pancakes, you will need speed of operating and/or a helper (much nicer to do these with a friend or member of the family!)

Put the flour and salt into a bowl and make a well in the centre. Pour in some of the milk and break the egg into this. Begin beating the mixture, adding the rest of the milk, then the water little by little until the batter is like thin cream.

Heat the pan with very little oil until the surface is coated with a thin film of oil. Pour in 2 - 3 tbsp of the batter, tipping the pan to allow the pancake mixture to cover the surface thinly. Initially use a higher heat until the white surface of the pancake bubbles and nearly dries (approx. 1-2 mins). Then flip with a spatula or toss the pancake and reduce the heat quickly. After 1-2 mins, turn the pancake onto the plate. Repeat the process whilst the pan is hot – a hot pan makes better pancakes! If you lack a helper, use what time you have to butter, sugar and lemon juice the cooked pancake, roll it up and store in a warm oven until all the pancakes are cooked.

Serve with lemon wedges or slices of fresh fruit and ice cream. Mmmm!

Chocolate and sweet potato cake

Sweet potato is a healthy food and reduces the amount of flour needed.
1 large or 2 medium sweet potatoes (or ordinary mashing potato), approx. 250g
100g / 2 tbsp chopped nuts, such as hazelnuts or walnuts
250g / 4-5 tbsp self-raising flour
50g / 2 oz / 2 tbsp cocoa powder
125 g polyunsaturated margarine
125 g caster sugar
2 eggs, lightly beaten
50 ml low fat milk (approx. half a cupful)
Pinch of salt

PREPARATION

Lightly grease a deep 20 cm cake tin. Preheat the oven to 1800C / Gas mark 4.

Peel and grate the sweet potato and mix with the flour, nuts, salt and cocoa. Cream together the margarine and sugar until light and fluffy. Gradually add the beaten eggs and milk. Fold in the chocolate potato mixture and transfer to the cake tin. Bake for 35 - 40 minutes or until cooked when tested with a skewer.

Use a low fat butter spread as a filling or icing or a fruity jam, marmalade or honey.

Date and Banana Cookies

75 g chopped dried dates
75 g finely chopped walnuts
3 medium bananas, mashed
175 g rolled oats
150 ml olive or sunflower oil
1 tsp vanilla essence

PREPARATION

Mix everything together really well. Put tablespoons of the mixture onto an oiled baking tray. Bake at gas mark 6 / 200°C for 15 - 20 mins until golden brown.

Epilogue

Once upon a time, I thought I would live a healthy life for another couple of decades or more. Then the CLL hit! I was knocked sideways by having to face an uncertain future.

Nine years on I am still here. I have experienced bad times as well as remission. I have been frightened, depressed, exhausted and sad. But during this time I have also been elated (at the birth of my grandchildren), happy to spend time with family and friends, done things I always wanted to do, and seen faraway places I only dreamed of before.

You too may have bad times but hang in there! Tomorrow is truly another day and the sun may shine for you. Good luck!

Max Ann McLaughlin de Boo

New Every Morning

Every day is a fresh beginning
Listen my soul to the glad refrain.
And, in spite of old sorrows
And older sinning,
Troubles forecasted
And possible pain,
Take heart with the day and begin again.

Susan Coolidge
(1835 - 1905)

References:
Helpful Organisations

Although these details were correct when the book was printed, some of them may have changed. If you have access to the internet it will be a simple matter to search for the organisation and check the contact details.

CancerBACUP
3 Bath Place, Rivington Street
London EC2A 3DR
Tel. 020 7696 9003
Freephone: 0808 800 1234
www.cancerbacup.org.uk

Leukaemia CARE
2, Shrubbery Avenue
Worcester, WR1 1QH
Tel. 01905 330 003
Email: support@leukaemiacare.org.uk

Cancer Research UK
PO Box 123, London WC2A
www.cancerhelp.org.uk

British Acupuncture Council
63, Jeddo Road, London W12 9HQ
Tel. 0208 735 0400
www.acupuncture.org.uk

British Association for Counselling
1, Regent Place, Rugby, Warwickshire CV21 2PJ
Tel. 0870 443 5232
www.counselling.co.uk and bacp@bacp.co.uk

British Wheel of Yoga
Central Office, 1 Hamilton Place, Boston Road
Sleaford, Lincs. NG34 7ES
Tel. 01529 306 851
www.bwy.org.uk

Disability Information and Services
Enquiry Line: 0800 882200

Disability Living Allowance & Attendance Allowance
08457 123456

International Federation of Professional Aromatherapists
82, Ashby Road, Hinckley, Leics. LE10 1SE
Tel. 01455 637 987
www.ifparoma.org

International Federation of Aromatherapists
www.int-fed-aromatherapy.co.uk

National Council of Psychotherapists
Tel. 0845 230 6072
www.natcouncilofpsychotherapists.org.uk

National Institute of Medical Herbalists
www.nimh.org.uk

National Register of Hypnosis and Psychotherapy
12, Cross Street, Nelson, Lancs. BB9 7EN
Tel. 0282 699 378
www.nrhp.co.uk

National Federation of Spiritual Healers (NFSH)
Old Manor Farm Studio, Church Street
Sunbury-on-Thames, Middlesex TW16 6RG
Tel. 0845 1232 777 (Ring for local branch information)
www.nfsh.org.uk

NHS Direct
Tel. 0845 4647
www.nhsdirect.nhs.uk

The Society of Homeopaths
11, Brookfield, Duncan Close
Northampton, NN3 6LW
Tel.0845 450 6611
www.homeopathy-soh.org

University of the Third Age (U3A)
Unit 3, Carpenters Court,
Bromley BR1 2RN
Tel. 0208 466 6139
Email: national.office@u3a.org.uk